Landscape with Moving Figures

A Decade on Dance

Laura Jacobs

Dance & Movement Press™

New York

Published in 2006 by Rosen Book Works, LLC.
Exclusively distributed by The Rosen Publishing Group, Inc., New York

Copyright © 2006 by Laura Jacobs

First edition

All rights reserved. No part of this book may be reproduced in any form without permission in writing from the publisher, except by a reviewer.

The essays in this volume previously appeared in the *New Criterion*. They have been slightly revised for this publication.

Interior book design by Jennifer Crilly

For more information regarding Dance & Movement Press, contact:
The Rosen Publishing Group, Inc.
29 East 21st Street
New York, NY 10010
1-800-237-9932
Visit our Web site at http://www.rosenpublishing.com
(select the Dance & Movement Press icon)

Library of Congress Cataloging-in-Publication Data

Jacobs, Laura A.
    Landscape with moving figures : a decade on dance / Laura Jacobs.— 1st ed.
    p. cm. — (Contemporary discourse on movement and dance)
    Includes index.
    ISBN 1-59791-001-5 (trade bdg.)
    1. Dance. I. Title. II. Series.

GV1617.J33 2006
792.8—dc22
                                                      2005023934

*To Jim,
and our three muses*

Table of Contents

Introduction 1

Promises, Promises (1995) 7
Figures in the Carpet (1996) 13
Milken on the Beach in China (1996) 21
Misha: Impossible (1997) 26
Frederick Ashton's England (1997) 32
Computer Games (1997) 41
Balanchine's Castle (1998) 47
Jerome Robbins Remembered (1998) 59
Tchaikovsky at the Millennium (1999) 64
Two Princes and a Mock Tudor (2000) 78
Taylor's Domain (2001) 87
Petipaw (2002) 94
How Good Is the Kirov? (2002) 103
Sellin' Out (2002) 115
Bubble Boy (2003) 120
Stromanizing (2004) 130
Assoluta (2004) 140

Index 154

Introduction

My earliest memory of dance is a color. When I was very young, my parents took my sister and me to a performance of *The Sleeping Beauty*. We sat high up in the balcony, and there my sister and I fought over a box of Raisinettes. I do not recall a step, a scene, a costume, but to this day I can still see the faraway glow of the stage, a hearth of lavender in the darkness.

Dance kept entering my life. There was the Christmas gift from a relative: a beautiful illustrated book called *The Stories of the Great Ballets*, and with it a 33 LP of *Les Sylphides* and *Sylvia*. The image on the record jacket was Degas' *Little Dancer of Fourteen Years*, wistful, historical, the totemic bronze of the statue at odds with the silvery orchestrations inside, an opposition that captured ballet's strange state of forever and never again. There was the night I stayed up late with my Aunt Cathi, who had herself been a dancer (the glamour!), to watch a movie called *The Red Shoes*. We watched it in the dark as if it were a horror film, and in some ways it is—you never forget those reds. There was another book, *The Golden Book of Ballet*. Holding onto the chair in my bedroom, I tried to teach myself positions from its pictures. Arabesque was the most seductive position of all: accomplishment, desire, caught and held in floating, flying, alignment. And with my parents there were more trips to the ballet, larger-than-life nights at the Civic Opera House of Chicago—women in diamonds, men in mink. I loved ballet. But as is often the case with girls, I loved horses more.

At sixteen I began to realize that riding wasn't going to be my life. It was then I decided to become a ballerina, simple as that. I knew it was a late start, so to save face I told everyone I was going

Introduction

to be a dance critic and needed to learn about dance from the inside out. My "critic" idea wasn't as out of the blue as it sounds. I knew about criticism from my father, a doctor who read music and movie reviews with delight, commented on them with brio, and urged his children to form their own opinions, to be able to explain why something was good or bad. These conversations with my father—at the table, in the car—were early lessons in how to debate and defend a work of art. It was he who one day said, as if he'd been considering it for some time, "I think you should be a fine-arts critic."

The weekly trip into Chicago for Saturday class at the Ruth Page Foundation—the *only* place to study, according to Aunt Cathi—soon became daily trips. The forty-minute train ride was part of the thrill. I was on my own, traveling to the land of artistry. And the rickety elevator up to the nineteenth floor with its crowded reception room and humid studio and ballet mothers knitting, always knitting, well, it was all too romantic. I had a natural turn-out and learned fast. Within a year I was in advanced class.

I continued dancing through freshman year at Vanderbilt University, then transferred to Northwestern so I could return to Ruth Page. Ballet gave me a rarefied other life, a mystique with prospective dates, and an escape from them as well. The mirror was not fooled. What I'd achieved was impressive but it wasn't enough and I'd never learned to spot. With graduation approaching, I decided to put my English degree to work. I would be a poet (no less), and for the next two years I wrote daily, feverishly, just as I had danced. The plan to be a critic was packed away with the pointe shoes.

And then it was unpacked. I started writing dance reviews for a Chicago paper because it paid real money; because having danced seriously I knew what I was talking about; and because the form, like poetry, was unbound, liberated, open to imaginative flight. You're working with something here and gone, living and vanished, concentrated and traceless. It was 1980, 1981, and the dance boom was still in swing. I'd been reading books by dancers since sixteen, but now I looked for critics. I discovered the pearls of Edwin Denby, the witty precision of Randall Jarrell. I sat up straight reading the stern sentences of Lincoln Kirstein. I happened upon Arlene Croce's *Afterimages*, and thought, Wow, a high-style way to write about dance. I didn't really have an end goal for my dance writing. I assumed I could never support myself with it and would always have to have a steady day job. My first real post—dance critic at the *Boston Phoenix*—was a plum made possible by nine-to-five Kelly Girl work. Nevertheless, I had a knack for the form, a fund of experience, and an eye to excel. I also had two inspiring editors: Kit Rachlis, who would cut my pieces into sections and reorganize them as drama; and Jeffrey Gantz, whose sharpened pencils taught me grammar and clarity. I learned how to write.

In 1983, darkness fell upon the decade and didn't lift. It was loss after loss, a series of disappearances, silent, momentous, history recorded in one's fingertips on the keyboard, and the heart still numb to that question: Who will replace? The giants, the geniuses who had shaped the dance landscape of the mid- to late-twentieth century, were dying. George Balanchine in 1983, Antony Tudor in 1987, Sir Frederick Ashton and Robert Joffrey in 1988, Alvin Ailey in 1989. Martha Graham and Agnes de Mille would live into the nineties (1991 and 1993), but were no longer doing important work. It was like the columns crumbling in *La Bayadère*. It was *Orpheus*: a glow receding, a narrow darkness taking them away. The giants who remained—Jerome Robbins, Paul Taylor, Merce Cunningham—were ever more precious. Meanwhile, the downtown scene was thriving, alive with talent, with young artists who might carry dance into the future. And then they too began dying. The AIDS epidemic was stalking the present and future of dance.

It wasn't stalking alone. The culture had changed. The trend of dumb-and-dumber had infected a media already addled on MTV cutting techniques, a literal break with linear thought, a nod to slasher sensibility. The high calling of high art was Greek to the grunge generation and a joke on Wall Street, where philanthropy was okay for Tom Wolfe's "lemon tarts" in Lacroix poof skirts but certainly not for the suits who bought up Chelsea, SoHo, and the Lower East Side, pricing out the very places where artists had lived, worked, rehearsed, and performed. Lottery replaced philan-

Introduction

thropy. And the new lottery mentality, winner take all, meant there was only enough goodwill—i.e., financial support—for one choreographer, one company, one vision, one dream . . . maybe three. So there was anger.

In 1994, that anger jumped beyond the world of dance into the currency of the culture. Bill T. Jones's *Still/Here*, a work about disease and the way the sick are marginalized, became the flash point for a divisive issue termed *victim art*. Arlene Croce struck the match when she "reviewed" the piece without seeing it. The writing was fiery, impassioned, but like fire it went in many directions, wherever there was wind and tinder. At the time I thought her review a rhetorical sensation. Reading it a few years later, I thought, It protests too much. There was something eerie in Croce's reaction to a dance with that title, as if it had hit a nerve, was holding up a mirror to her own diminishing presence in the pages of *The New Yorker*. *Still/Here*? It was hard to tell. Are you "here" if you won't go to the performance? And what if—and this is the case with so many balletomanes weaned on Balanchine—nothing you see eases your pain at his passing? Croce's floating away (in a bubble or on a broomstick, colleagues were of two minds) left the landscape unsupervised in a way it hadn't been for decades.

I've begun this collection with my review of *Still/Here* because it is nonsense to say something is unreviewable, and because this dance about presence and absence is a marker, a monument to a landscape where the comfortable old assumptions, expectations, don't play anymore. To write seriously about dance through the nineties and into this new century has itself been an act of "still/here." Dance as an art has been victimized by funding cuts. Dance as an exhilarating communal experience is at odds with a culture addicted to PlayStations and computer screens. And our loss of the greatness we once took for granted—and what a luxury that was—is still painful to the touch. I recently watched the Robert Wise-Jerome Robbins film of *West Side Story*, maligned today because a new generation of critics accepts Pauline Kael's damning judgment as if it were wine and wafer. I was mesmerized by the beginning—silence that was already a form of dance—and speechless when the film ended.

It wasn't just the ripping choreographic energy, and a blazing score that screams with strength, and a cinematic construction kinetically engaged. It was this gang of talent, these elbowing egos driving as one: Bernstein, Robbins, Laurents, Sondheim. Will we ever see such a wealth of talent again? Do we have a society that even wishes it, or could recognize it, or would support it?

I became dance critic at the *New Criterion* in that year of 1994. Then, as now, there were only a handful of periodicals in America that covered dance in essay form, half a handful in lengths over five thousand words. The *New Criterion* was one of them. Editors Hilton Kramer and Roger Kimball were eager to cover dance seriously, and they wanted as many essays as I could write. It was as if they'd given me wings. Indeed, to write generously about dance in this era of diminishment, I myself would have to bring more to the stage: more memories, more insight from the days of my own dance aspirations, more of the wisdom that illuminates intermission chat, more of my life outside the theater. At the *New Criterion* I began to write about dance my way. The performances reviewed in this book date from 1994 to 2004.

In 1994 I took up, as well, a pursuit somewhat opposite to the red-and-gold rhythm of the theater, and that was birdwatching. Over the years the promenade, the lobby, can get tricky with the agendas of peers and their shifting alliances, stuffy with works you've seen too many times. The act of going outdoors to look for whatever nature might send into sight was refreshing, calling on a concentration similar to that of watching a dance, yet requiring no response other than wonder. The privilege of stumbling upon something alien, wordless, priceless; the challenge of identifying it; the sharpening of one's eyes, the quickening of one's instincts—I was able to bring this solitary seeing back to the theater. I found myself writing with a new sense of space, a trust that my essays didn't have to begin at 8 P.M. but could drop into the landscape strategically, fancifully, landing in first position at the barre or in an old photograph never forgotten. These beginnings forced new paths and vistas upon me, and sometimes leaps.

At its best, criticism is a performance too. Hence the title of this book, *Landscape with Moving Figures*. It makes me think of a Martha

Introduction

Graham dance. Or it could be a ballet, very Jerry. When you walk alone into a forest or meadow there is a sense that you've slipped beyond an invisible curtain into another world. Dance is like that. As Leonardo da Vinci wrote, "Movement is the cause of all life." In these essays I've tried to slip beyond the curtain, to identify what is alive there, what is endangered, and what is moving.

Promises, Promises

It's never been much fun writing about choreography by Bill T. Jones. It was easier when he worked with Arnie Zane, co-founder of the dance company they shared. Jones was tall, black, and statuesque and Zane was short, white, and weasely. Neither was a born dancer with a born dance body and the work they did together was like a Hope and Crosby road movie: they made it up as they went along—posturing, pontificating, parodying. It was two guys who knew nothing about making dances making dances. Zane was the better mover; quick, sly, a sort of dance-department pickpocket, wedges and squiggles pinched from the air. Jones was lumbering, lagging behind, his lumpy muscles somehow in the way. The two-some was openly gay, and soon had a following that was looking for an alternative dance by alternative dancers. Their biggest hit together was called *Secret Pastures* (1984), a Frankenstein story in which Jones was the fabricated man, Zane the feisty scientist. I remember *Pastures* as zany, apolitical, a parable of the ways the dance-illiterate Jones was being honed for civilization.

And zoned too. Because in the years since *Pastures* had its premiere at the Brooklyn Academy of Music (BAM), since Zane died of AIDS in 1988 and Jones himself announced he was HIV-positive, Jones has continued to work in a territory of experiment. Citing "dogma" as the stifling signifier of the dance scene, he has remained on purpose dance-illiterate. You might describe him as amateur avant-garde. Though he moves better than he used to, the pieces he choreographs still look like they were made by a beginner who took from books what you can only learn by doing. Wearing his defiance like a chasuble, he has emerged as a sort of footlights preacher-man, complete with growls and pounces, sexed-up genuflections, a curling lip behind totemic masks. Pushing hot buttons in the manner of Madonna, that self acknowledged legislator of the world, Jones makes work that attempts to rattle us out of our complacency—he's a shake-down shaman. Humming hostility is the energy he brings to the stage, and brooding quiet. He's more interesting when standing still or giving curtain speeches than when moving. And a mean curtain speech goes a long way these days.

The press release announcing December's BAM performances of *Still/Here* began, "1994 could be called the year of Bill T. Jones," and indeed the press kit was crammed with four-color clips, cover stories, and—drum roll—a gigantic puffball of a *New Yorker* preview piece by Henry Louis Gates, Jr., which may have set a new precedent for highbrow hype, and most certainly triggered Arlene Croce's brilliant blast at hype's circling satellites: victim art, the grants game, our TV nation. Sifting through the press material was more like watching MacNeil/Lehrer than reading about dance. Tasteful reporting, plaintive political summation, cultural context, profile information—but where was *Still/Here*? There were descriptions of the dance in workshop, of what happens onstage, and actual lines of text that are heard or sung. But a formal sense of the dance itself? It seems that other critics aren't having fun writing about choreography by Bill T. Jones either.

Jones's star rose in the same decade as Mark Morris's, and there are similarities between the two dancers in sexual orientation and chest-pounding irreverence and even, curiously, the use of sign language in their work. But Morris was never above or irreverent about craft. He learned to stitch steps in the master tradition, and while the later work often disappointed (especially after similar BAM media gluts), the early excitement of seeing dances built from the floor up, having an acute coherence and an almost divine spark of time and place, was honestly won. Jones, meanwhile, was still cracking eggs. He never picked up the rudiments of the *enchaînement*—the linking of steps into a phrase—or cared to understand how a phrase becomes an articulation, an image, a shape within a rhythm, a vision within a shape that you can actually remember and play over in your mind and call a dance. Perhaps he was too interested in talking his ideas.

Morris could spin out *enchaînements* in his sleep, and he took as his cues not only music but also text to music. He leaned on these too heavily. But do not underestimate an audience's pleasure in "association" or the way an artist learns to refine and nuance such blunt beginnings. When Morris used signing or made visual pictures that mimed a libretto, you saw the layering technique and felt the cognitive tension between two dimensions (abstract language and the concrete body), which thickened and quickened the dance and pointed to more sophisticated expression down the road. Jones's sign language is without correspondences to any other vocabulary, makes no visual associations (think Jodie Foster's Nell). It's an obtuse semaphore system of hand shapes and gestures, often accompanied by discussions that sound like Karen Finley in a quizzical mood. The dances wear a gloss of huffing, puffing intent and are performed with a professional gleam. "At least *he* must know what he's doing," you think as you sink into your seat.

With all the flurry of hyperbole surrounding *Still/Here*, the hosannas in *Newsweek* and reports of foot-stomping audiences in Lyon, I went to BAM thinking, okay, maybe it's a breakthrough. The last Jones piece performed there had been *Last Supper at Uncle Tom's Cabin/The Promised Land*—a typical Jones/Zane title in its hip conflation of too many ideas, its persecution complex, and its outsized scale of effort. What I remember of that evening, again, is not a dance (actually, not even a step) but a pileup of theatrical strategies, chief among them Jones wandering through asking ethical questions of a priest. *Last Supper* was really a kind of happening. It climaxed with a stream of naked dancers, running and bouncing, showing us their . . . equality . . . how, with our clothes off, we are all naked.

Still/Here takes place in the same pseudo-philosophical space as *Last Supper*, only its community is vulnerable in a different way: it is mortality we share, and don't you forget it. For this piece Jones set up workshops around the country in which he talked to people who had diseases from which they would probably not recover. Tapes from these workshops are arranged into an aural score, spliced into gray chamber music, and lines from the tapes have been elaborated into urgent songs sung live by gravel-voiced Odetta.

Landscape with Moving Figures

The first half of the dance, "Still," presents the dancers as characters from the tapes: each comes forward and strikes defining poses, a sort of valiant voguing. Then, to voices discussing diagnosis, denial, and "slash, poison, or burn" as treatment choices, dancers tackle one another to show the assault of illness, or engage in reaching-out gestures of comfort and sympathy, a Hallmark ritual that strains both eye and mind.

Incessant video business by Gretchen Bender provides something to look at once you realize that Jones's choreography hasn't developed a jot. It's his own memory-defying, anti-dance dogma—the parade of poses, the belligerent squats and karate kicks worked into depthless lines across the stage. Cobalt-blue screens glow in the dark; speeded-up slide shows of diseased body parts flash in grotesque REM spectacles; filmed images of dancers are distorted to make them look like spreading solar systems; identical medical-book drawings of pink hearts beat on five screens. It's a high-tech checkup, your own personal future shock (prognosis poor). In the evening's second part, "Here," the movement is pitched higher. The body parts flash faster. The lighting goes a garish yellow, and a video monitor is wheeled in, Jones's face on the screen (his only appearance in *Still/Here*). The evening ends in an orgy of heavy-metal squalling, the dancers wildly circling Jones's screen image, a talking head saying nothing.

The promised land. It was part of the title of Jones's last big piece, and the idea recurs here in this final shot of dancers revelling round their boob-tube Aaron, waiting for the word that doesn't come. The one true moment in the evening, it reminds me of the promise held out through Tony Kushner's *Angels in America*, the secret future that the angel is going to impart, but in six hours of stage time never does because Kushner's arguments alone can't take us there—the writing has to do that, and, like Jones, technically he's not up to it. Art does tell truths and secrets, but rarely in big block letters, clever rant, or video speechifying. Meanings are folded into textures, into the flights and private follies of an advancing technique, and into moments that are structured strongly enough that we can recall them as phenomena, as places in nature.

I think of Paul Taylor's *Company B*, a hit from 1991 set to light,

10

jazzy, jiggly wartime tunes by the Andrews Sisters—songs now slick with nostalgia. Working in the jitterbug idioms of the forties, Taylor spins out dazzling variations on the theme of love as war, a metaphor expressing the violence of desire, the race against time, men falling and falling again. The dance is a pop romp, yet through the use of silhouette and slow motion in the background, elegy filters in, creating a dark zone "over there." And then Taylor crosses the threshold to another over-there. In the dance "I Can Dream, Can't I," behind an agitated solo for one woman, two men move in mirror step, a backdrop to her longing, a soldierly frieze. For only a second one of them half-turns to fully face the other, and in that nearly missable second, so effortlessly achieved and dramatically fine, the dance is charged, completed in the present tense. It's a different dance now, not about then but always, the daily destructions born boisterously in our blood.

I also think of Neil Greenberg's *Not-About-AIDS-Dance*, which was performed last May at The Kitchen and repeated there in December. An attempt to make art that holds hard formally, acknowledging a dire diagnosis and a stream of dying friends without getting lost in loss, Greenberg presents a work of unrelenting, interlocking, deep-lunged dance. Costumed in spartan white shorts and tops, situated in a duskily lit black-box space, the only props a naked branch and a sword, the piece is wintry, isolated, yet heated with concentration, hurtling forward. On the back wall white titles, sometimes witty, tell of events, fears, and deaths that happened during the making of the dance. The only backward glance occurs when Greenberg arranges himself into a careful picture, behind him the words, "This is how my brother Jon looked in a coma." The intimacy of the moment is stabbing, an ache moated by the abstraction around it, ennobled by Greenberg's classical stance, its echo through centuries of premature deaths. Months later, this spare dance stands clearer and taller in memory, like white marble columns, an ode to stoicism.

Mass dying of the young is a new subject for our time, but it is not a new subject historically, nor has it always been expressed literally. One of the great "march on" dances of the century is Sir Frederick Ashton's *Symphonic Variations*, a strange work that Ashton plotted while in the RAF. Having plunged into mysticism during the war (St. Theresa of Avila, St. John of the Cross), Ashton came back to the Sadler's Wells studio with an eccentric four-seasons scenario sketched to music by César Franck (a sentence from Part 4: "Art and Faith united in one unseverable bond"). The ballet emerged, however, as a plotless work for six dancers. The backdrop was lemony green, a swooping curve that might be an enlarged site on a relief map, and the dancers' white tunics and headpieces suggested sylvan sculptures come to life—*veritas* in toe shoes.

Technically painstaking, the ballet calls for rushes of raw strength checked within pristine, almost antiquated stanzas—you might call it a rite of spring inside a requiem. *Symphonic Variations*'s syntactical precision seems, for Ashton anyway, a kind of life itself, art's answer to disaster. You want to see it again immediately, to reread that language, return to that unity. Watching an aggressive muddle like *Still/Here*, you'd rather make a break for it. We're all going to suffer and die is its one-note refrain. And that we already knew.

February 1995

Figures in the Carpet

One of the basic poses in ballet, arabesque takes its name from a form of Moorish ornament. In ballet it is a position of the body, in profile, supported on one leg . . . with the other leg extended behind and at right angles to it, and the arms held in various harmonious positions creating the longest possible line from the fingertips to the toes. The shoulders must be held square to the line of direction.
—Technical Manual and Dictionary of Classical Ballet

The arabesque looks simple at first: a storklike standing on one leg, the other leg arrowed straight back, a banner, a comet's tail. The arabesque is odd (which explains the mixed metaphor in the previous sentence). It is complex, a pulse point of oppositions: vertical versus horizontal, stillness versus flight. And it is subject to strict rules. The above-cited dictate about the shoulders—that they must be held square—is much like the fairy godmother in *Cinderella* saying, Leave by midnight. The image dissolves when the rules are broken.

Arabesque is the queen of ballet steps, its own rule. That long line from fingertips to toe is a kind of horizon, a sovereignty surveyed. It can even seem a flying carpet, the dancer's torso riding up above the earth. Among the lost Balanchine ballets most mourned by the late Lincoln Kirstein was *The Figure in the Carpet* from the 1960s, a work whose dances, he wrote, "suggested the age in which the arabesque of Islamic ornament wove itself into Western European fashion and design, just as the arabesque, our ballet position, fixed the place of Islam in a royal academy of dancing at

Versailles." Kirstein remarks that *The Figure in the Carpet* "was too unwieldy to maintain"; others suggest it was musically monotonous. Arabesques, too, are prey to such failings. This statuesque design can quickly become heavy, static. As *The Oxford Companion to Art* reminds us, the arabesque was abstracted from a plant form. It must breathe and grow.

And so the great arabesques are more than a pose, they are a phenomenon, like Caruso's ringing high C or Montserrat Caballé's stratospheric pianissimo. They can suggest the high wire, held note of a violin; or silence within a soliloquy, that stirring in the shadow of language (another kind of held note). In fact, arabesques actually do cast shadows. And as George Balanchine showed in his 1928 *Apollo*, they are like rays of sun.

Dancers need not think about the arabesque in such fanciful terms. They learn by example, trying on the signature arabesques of ballerinas, no two alike. And they fight for their own arabesque: the lift in the leg, the hold in the spine, the continuous, coursing energy required to keep the toe pointed and the shoulders from slipping open like a loose door. They fight to keep the arabesque alive. A good arabesque never gets easy.

And a great one is unforgettable. Margot Fonteyn's—unembellished, never higher than her hip, but not giving an inch of what it had—was English iconography. Moira Shearer's really did look like a leap from a balcony (she of *The Red Shoes* fame). On film, the Kirov's Natalia Dudinskaya shows a power forging through the pelvis that is practically continental, like the coming of cold. Irina Kolpakova of the next generation? Her light, slim, big arabesque was a maiden's search through silver birches. And let's not forget Gelsey Kirkland's diminutive, driven arabesque (she who wrote *Dancing on My Grave*): taut, fraught, her pink toe-tip dipped in curare.

Suzanne Farrell's arabesque embodied an era (the Farrell era). Huge, unforced, eternally new-looking, it could be cool and blinding—blizzard white—or balmy, a white night. You could live in it if you had to. After Farrell retired, Maria Calegari carried the flame—a small golden one compared to Farrell's blue flare. Calegari reminded me of a dictionary drawing of the parabola, her lifted leg taking its momentum from the tensile U in the small of her back. When she performed that stationary, hand-turned arabesque in Balanchine's *Serenade*, her persimmon hair down around her shoulders, her arabesque rising like a tightening bow, she was goddess Diana securing a cliff top. Kyra Nichols, who is now the reigning ballerina at New York City Ballet, has everything but a memorable arabesque. Perhaps that is why her command has been so retiring, so lacking in ceremony.

Where are the great arabesques? That is the question that slowly formed this spring, expanding to fill the empty space left by the season's handful of banal new ballets. At NYCB, Peter Martins can no longer make a choreographic ripple. His ballets, whatever the idiom, are increasingly unmusical and indistinct; divorced, it feels, from warm-blooded classicism (they're test-tube ballets). Kevin O'Day, a former Twyla Tharp dancer who has been a quick hit as a choreographer, makes aggressive little Gen X dances, Calvin Klein ads dressed in glam black and trapped in a kaleidoscope. As with this season's *Badchonim* ("Merrymakers"), they wow the audience with their zip and symmetry but require no commitment at all from the dancers. At American Ballet Theatre, the revolving door spun and swept Jiri Kylian back into the Metropolitan Opera House with a New Age, or Old Egypt, ritual called *Stepping Stones*—solemn, sinewy, po-mo, pompous. There was also a new Tharp wiggle-world, *The Elements*, and a pretty but inconsequential production of *Cinderella*, borrowed from the Houston Ballet.

The companies didn't play up the premieres. Their focus was on young dancers—new girls and star boys. And anyway, one no longer expects a communicative piece of choreography. Premieres post-Balanchine haven't been hot events since Baryshnikov left ABT, Mark Morris plateaued, and Twyla Tharp turned into her own bowl-cut cottage industry. Debuts are what's left. High hopes get pinned to kids barely out of the academy, young things from the School of American Ballet or the Ukraine. Premature hopes. This year, the NYCB "It girl" is Maria Kowroski. At ABT, it's Paloma Herrera.

Maria Kowroski was already talked about last year, but she broke into important roles this spring, receiving raves. I went time and again to figure out what the fuss was about and saw a very long-legged, very loose-jointed dancer with rather glassy good looks. In a performance of *Symphony in C*—the jewel-box second movement—Kowroski was like melting taffy, overextended and going weak. Was this a clueless performance or a terrified one? By her first attempt at Terpsichore (in *Apollo*), Kowroski had pulled herself together and marked through the ballet without incident. I say "marked" because she wasn't exactly dancing, she was getting the steps right. Unhinged again in *The Prodigal Son*, Kowroski's Siren slam-danced the poor Prodigal.

Kowroski will improve. She will learn to get through ballets in one piece. She has an instrument. What one doesn't see is technique invested with a personality. Indeed, Kowroski's arabesque is a rubbery type that is increasingly the norm at NYCB. (Is it becoming state of the art?) A trombone slide into height that's out of sync with a composed whole, this arabesque has no interior opposition and therefore no dynamics—it's a trick arabesque. The perennially promising Margaret Tracey and the double-jointed Diana White are of a kind with Kowroski. These are big arabesques, way above hip level, but they are not good ones. An antidote arabesque came in *Who Cares?* It was the parallel-to-ground, swift spear of senior ballerina Merrill Ashley (Who cares? She cares!). Complete clarity is more impressive than automatic height.

Compared to Kowroski, the raven-haired, twenty-year-old Argentinean, Paloma Herrera, is vividly present, and she really does have a textbook technique. Her proportions are as perfect as Kowroski's, though on a smaller scale—short yet supple from waist to shoulder, extra long from hip to toe—and she has a strength that rarely accompanies these proportions. Furthermore, she's a textbook drawing in three dimensions; there's a sense of curve and volume in her dancing, a palpable roundness in her head-on attack. Her long arched pointes grab ground like talons. I liked Herrera better as a budding soloist, when she had more glow and desire, as well as more weight. Now, catapulted to the top of the roster, it's as if she's set her jaw and locked her mind.

One of the few gifts Herrera was not granted is an easy smile, though it used to be easier and more charming. As Kitri in *Don Quixote*, she was in a snit rather than high spirited, grudgingly happy. Trying to live up to her star status, she punctuates heavily, selling stunts when she should be exploring the music (even bad music). Like a slot machine hitting the jackpot, Herrera hits her balances with a *ker-chink!*, holding them through wobble and sway in an exaggerated vibrato, sending the audience weirdly wild. In this she was abetted by partners who are right for her in stature (Julio Bocca, Angel Corella) but wrong in spirit. If Herrera has the potential to be more than a Technique Machine—which is what ABT's Susan Jaffe has become, having been given the same rush in her ingenue years—she should be allowed to find out now, not goaded into circus work with Tasmanian Devils in dance belts. The modest, plummy, loving performance she gave four seasons ago in Ashton's *Symphonic Variations* is a kind of dancing now lost to her.

But as spring progressed there were signs of return. Midseason, Herrera did not oversell her solo in the Rose Adagio from *The Sleeping Beauty*, a part built around balances on pointe, and her *Tchaikovsky Pas de Deux* with Corella grew lighter, more musically spontaneous. And throughout the whole season, even during the most discouraging grandstanding, there was Herrera's arabesque—undeniably superb, utterly dependable, a lush physics that might have been devised by Oppenheimer in a moment of whimsy. Julie Kent, of the Wedgwood beauty, the couturish bones and pale tones, is more inventive than Herrera. Amanda McKerrow is more refined. But neither has an arabesque that can compete with Herrera's for might, security, the infrastructural play of opposing forces, curves sprung tight inside angles. Kent's inconsistency in this step—her arabesque line large and ecstatic in *Romeo and Juliet*, brittle and smack up against her limitations in *Swan Lake*—spoke to her technical inconsistency all around, a disappointment in a dancer with so much imagination. McKerrow's season was simply off, her arabesque rarely square, authority slipping out the door. But Herrera's arabesque, it kept bringing me back to her and to the question: Will it ever be the summation of an expressive whole?

That kind of arabesque belonged to but one person this season, a man, ABT's Vladimir Malakhov. For possibly the first time in this century, men's arabesques were more compelling than women's (I'm thinking also of NYCB's Ethan Stiefel and Igor Zelensky). The spring 1996 season in general belonged to the men; Lincoln Center could have flown a flag tagged "Where the Boys Are." And ballet management played up the testosterone. Balanchine's nod to masculine splendor, *Apollo*—with its big, juicy, heroic role was in repertory at both NYCB and ABT, an unusual occurrence. Many men danced it, though rarely more than once (leaving no chance for skill to build). Still it was fascinating to see such a variety of types chisel into that ice-white iconography. As if to stress the tipping scales between gender, a program conflict cropped up early in the season, leaving the unhappy choice: Julie Kent at ABT in Tudor's *The Leaves Are Fading* or Ethan Stiefel at NYCB in *Apollo*. These were long-awaited debuts for both dancers. With Stiefel soon to leave NYCB for a European company, I went to *Apollo*. Quite reasonably, another critic I know chose Kent *because* Stiefel was leaving, rendering his performance "an experiment in a void."

When I first came to care about classical dance, I paid no attention to male dancers. Ballet was turn-out and toe shoes, and women had both. Men, with their tighter, narrower pelvises, could hardly muster half as much rotation in the hips, and of course didn't go on pointe. By college I did care about male dancers. Rudolf Nureyev was a household name, and Mikhail Baryshnikov had just defected. But even then, I only loved Rudi for his love of ballet. Because men didn't have the turn-out, they just didn't have the territory of women—the poetic power. Baryshnikov, plush in turn-out, with a stately, plump arabesque, was the exception that proved the rule.

In the persons of Vladimir Malakhov and Ethan Stiefel, however, we are now seeing male dancing based on a fully rotated and integrated, almost female turn-out. When male strength meets such technical refinement the result is jaw-dropping clarity—a kind of enchantment. Stiefel is never better than in magic-forest ballets like *Valse Fantaisie*, *A Midsummer Night's Dream*, and *The Sleeping Beauty* Act Two; in roles of classical scale this smallish dancer seems to grow a foot, phrasing daringly, leaving the limits of tradition behind. His arabesque is ardent. In more prosaically scaled work (Robbins, Martins) Stiefel can seem slight, under-engaged. He needs classicism.

And Malakhov. When you first see this dancer set foot upon the stage, though blond and not overly muscled, you can't help thinking of Nureyev. He has the deliberate walk and the stage-bound self-containment. When he enters for the balcony scene of *Romeo and Juliet*, the cape is redundant—he's already caped in concentration. Clive Barnes called him a "Rudi wannabe," sarcasm that missed the larger point. Malakhov is more important for the ways he's unlike Rudi. Where Nureyev brought dark force to his dancing, Malakhov brings lightness, restraint. Where Nureyev dragged sexuality into the picture, Malakhov can seem beyond it. And unlike Nureyev, he's not out to conquer classical technique, he's in league with it. He can break your heart with a *tendu*.

Malakhov has feet any female would be pleased with; his demi-pointe (work on tiptoe) is sensitive, springy, fascinatingly feline. Heading into a leap he gets finer, feathery, lofting off the ball of his foot—not heavier as most men do. In every step Malakhov shows you the interior logic of ballet technique, its unique system of torsion, leverage, and lift. Not only does he have quintessentially pure "placement" (the solar plexus properly positioned over the hips), he enunciates through the torso with amazing equilibrium and nuance, bracing brazenly back into big air moves (as only Misha did), and calibrating balances so that they look like expressions of idealism. This fluid and articulate discipline gives Malakhov a special phosphorescence. He glows in the dark. And I like the way Malakhov has absorbed both Nureyev and Baryshnikov into his system—making for yet another electric opposition. When Malakhov's onstage, everyone stands up straighter, high on his high.

There are those who feel Malakhov's best move is his grand jeté, and in his body it is a thing of surreal beauty. Soaring in a perfect split, he has a particularly arresting way of floating at the top—a countertenor who's hit his zone—suspending the moment with a gentle gesture of the palms, as if silencing the sky. Still, I think his alabaster arabesque comes first. Partly there's the shock of seeing it on a man. Partly there is Malakhov's deep belief in it. This arabesque has aura—an Apollonian symmetry and sensation of ascent (the arabesque design, it turns out, first appeared in Hellenistic times).

And yet, despite what would seem to be a natural fit, Malakhov, and Stiefel as well, looked disconnected from the role of Apollo, as if technique was getting in the way. It is well known that Balanchine viewed his Apollo as a rough young god. The role was choreographed for Serge Lifar, a rough young Russian with not much turn-out or finish. The man who commanded the role of Apollo this season was Igor Zelensky, a large, rough-hewn dancer with a mountain-range arabesque, big and simple, and upper-body strength to burn. The audience still prefers this kind of macho, and in the first round of Apollos, I preferred Zelensky, too. The Siberian size of him was moving.

Apollo is an allegory about the making of a dancer, an artist, and the centrality of *Apollo* this season is an allegory in its own right. In this ballet, man is the center of the universe; women are handmaid, mother, or muse. The ballerina role of Terpsichore is equal to Apollo's, but only if the dancer makes it so, and none did. It is a curious time in classical dance when men seem the center of its universe, when women are stuck while men are evolving. What could account for this? Well, to the novice audience, male virtuosity is a good deal more accessible than female. It's certainly easier to market. Hence the hyping of that little twister Angel Corella, an eager talent, too eagerly sacrificing alignment for bravura. More insidiously, it is easier for today's choreographers to create for men. Men don't have the female's historical/metaphorical baggage (they were never handmaids, mothers, or muses), men don't possess that parallel universe—pointe. Twyla Tharp, for example, reconstituted her cloying ballet from last year, *Americans We*, by upping the masculinity quotient and dropping Corella into its center. Now it's whiz-bang rousing. Her new ballet, *The Elements*, comes suddenly into focus whenever men take center stage. Women are too complicated, caught in limbo between a rich poeticized past and the meaningless postmodern moment. What do ballerinas want? I used to feel I knew. What's missing? Choreographers who care about arabesque.

September 1996

Milken on the Beach in China

Just minutes into Karole Armitage's *The Predators' Ball: Hucksters of the Soul*—her new multimedia theater piece presented at the Brooklyn Academy of Music in October—I couldn't stop thinking of that strange, hothouse creature of the forties and fifties, the dream ballet. These fifteen-minute "ballets," the expression of a character's dream or fantasy, pinpointed the show's inner conflict and poeticized it. They worked within the Broadway musical as the show's high-art cadenza, a wordless tour de force. And they reflected the Freudian analysis that was de rigueur with the literary set, not to mention neurotic Broadway types, in mid-twentieth-century America. Couched late in the show, surrealistically staged and often sophomorically symbolic, dream ballets were little landscapes of the subconscious: an epiphany inside a pirouette. Recreated in the movie versions of Broadway shows, the ballets were opened up, filmed on vast sound stages—ninety parts sky to ten parts people—as if to stress the unrealness of the dream, its atmosphere of gravity without weight. It is on film, in fact, in movies like *Oklahoma!*, *Carousel*, *An American in Paris*, and *Singin' in the Rain*, that most of us saw our first dream ballet. It had become a deep pocket in a celluloid strip.

I was thinking of the dream ballet because so much of what now passes for storytelling on the stage is not actual narrative but the fifteen-minute dream ballet expanded to fill a two- to three-hour time slot. BAM's Next Wave Festival specializes in this species of theater—has been actively breeding it for fourteen years. The big bang, of course, was *Einstein on the Beach*. The big flop, *Endangered Species* (the title referring less to the animals forced into postmodern posturing than to the theater as we once knew it).

In its progressive programming, BAM has actively sought and supported works of performance art or *Tanztheater* or dreamscape or "opera" (quotation marks built-in), pieces unmoored from genre, defying categorization. The spacey, irradiated picturings of Robert Wilson's stage, the circle of hairy hell that is an evening with Pina Bausch, the aggressive abstracts of Anna Teresa de Keersmaeker, Martha Clarke's morphing narratives—it's a theater of dreamy, free, often too free, association. Even the operas, usually composed by Philip Glass (*Einstein on the Beach*, the recent Cocteau trilogy) or John Adams (*Nixon in China*, *The Death of Klinghoffer*), their loop music scores gliding like a tracking shot without end, spin forth as film from a reel. At BAM, it's as if the film form of the dream ballet had been airmailed back to the East Coast stage, complete with a sprocketed sense of the void. Weightless gravity is alive and well in New York City.

"I wanted to make a kind of post-MTV production where image and a cinematic style could tell a story with all this kind of dance and movement around it." That's Karole Armitage talking about *The Predators' Ball*, her post-MTV dreamscape evocation of the rise and fall of leveraged buyout king Michael Milken.

Armitage is a BAM baby. Though her early choreography was presented in New York's downtown spaces where, doing a poststructuralist turn as Suzanne Farrell, she found her supersophisticated following, Armitage's later work premiered at BAM. It was the eighties, and she was flush with a Guggenheim, a famous fiancé (David Salle, who also had a Guggenheim—how's that for matching grants?), a commission from Baryshnikov at American Ballet Theatre, hip clothes and a punk hairdo (or punk clothes and a hip hairdo), and—talk about having it all—friendship with the Material Girl herself, Madonna. And she tried to put it all on the stage. As early as *The Mollino Room* for ABT you could see that the Salle presence in her work had a deadening effect; the sourball backdrops he did for her dances were pure pose and attitude, no give. But Salle was cultural capital, and he remained a big influence in her two-act work that premiered at BAM in 1987, *The Elizabethan Phrasing of Albert Ayler*.

Pointe shoes in film dream ballets, especially when the shoes were in Technicolors other than pink, always smacked of the exotic, a self-conscious artiness. And that's how Karole Armitage has always worn her pointes—as if the camera were running. *Elizabethan Phrasing* was really more of a home movie than a ballet, a séance in the living room, object lessons floating by: here's our jazz pics, our fifties furnishings, our flea market/art market classicism, our cultural cachet (or was it cachepots?). In the *New Criterion*, February 1988, Jed Perl pointed out the acquisitive nature of the Armitage/Salle sensibility. No wonder they're attracted to Milken.

The one thing Armitage couldn't do, and it became more apparent with every premiere, was "extend classicism"—everybody's misguided mission in ballet post-Balanchine. Souping it up with SoHo symbolism, girding up in black leather, cracking a whip while doing the *développés* of one of Balanchine's bacchantes, Armitage didn't look bad (rather, she looked *baaaaad, man*). Still it was always the Karole Armitage Show, not classical expression evolved but a commentary on where that expression was forced to go kicking and screaming. If Suzanne Farrell dancing Balanchine was a story within a story (woman as dream ballet), Armitage dancing Armitage was lipstick on the mirror, kisses to the cognoscenti.

The funny thing about *The Predators' Ball* is that it doesn't even look like Karole Armitage but like BAM. When young Michael Milken scribbles mathematical formulas on a blackboard, I found myself thinking of *Einstein on the Beach*. And that keening kind of not-quite-aria, not-quite-recetitive singing—it's so *Nixon in China* (in the role of Milken, Thomas Jay Ryan looks and sounds compellingly like Nixon). The video screen that was rolled onstage from time to time worked its own déjà vu: Bill T. Jones's *Still/Here* was still here. (Put a screen onstage and people will strain to watch that screen, no matter how small, instead of the live performers.)

As for Armitage's choreography, it has finally succumbed to the nineties norm, what might be called post-perspective classicism. This is ballet that uses classical steps but without any real feeling for the interior space of the stage, its invisible but formidable tiers and topographies. The result is an incessant chorus-line look, rows of synchronized movement with punched-up dynamics, or simple kicks in canon. The only way to get crescendo out of such flat composition is either to throw more dancers on the stage or to fake the effect with speed and stretch, a kind of dancing in extremis. William Forsythe and Peter Martins are the main practitioners of PPC, and Armitage has joined the club. When she introduces a lone girl who bourrées and balances in a white unitard—Idealism! Hope!—it's so out of context it's corny. Extending classicism may no longer be Karole's concern, but when did she go tone-deaf?

I notice that I haven't described the show yet. Score: a mix of fashion-show music (i.e., Eurodisco) and poignant symphonic by Georges Delerue. Lighting: Palladium dark, dank, with neon highlights—Wall Street awake at 4 A.M. Costumes: predominantly suits and suspenders (great looking in full-corps scenes). Narrative strategy no. 1: scenes built on symbols, such as the section about Milken's X-shaped conference table (dancers made X signs with their arms and legs), or the almost exciting sequence of Ron Perelman's hostile takeover of Revlon, symbolized by supermodels (the scene accumulates well, but goes nowhere). Narrative strategy no. 2: name that echo. Who's the guy in the silver suit? Thyades, a Caliban-type sprite. What are those weird chairs with telephones? Quotrons, designed as if by Kandinsky. Who does that insinuating voice-over sound like? HAL, the computer from *2001: A Space Odyssey*.

Reviewers noted that although the show didn't add up to much it was always lively. Is keeping the audience distracted the same as drawing it in? Considering how fast the show moved, it was surprising how soon into each scene one's attention flagged. Armitage's quick cutting wasn't always MTV-quick enough. The actual ballroom scene, which came near the end of the show and might have been a glittering and meticulous coup de théâtre, was a sloppy letdown. Costumed in high-court French decadence, it predictably devolved into a tacky orgy.

At the end of a long voice-over in which HAL details the genius of young Michael Milken, he finally says: "If you could get inside the head of a genius what would you find? You would find nothing at all—because you don't speak the language." This is a good summation of *The Predators' Ball*. Inside its lightboard of flashes, gimmicks, impressions, suggestions, projections, and tableaux, there is finally nothing at all. That nothing is not what's missing from Milken, it's about Armitage: she doesn't have a language. In the days when she was trying to speak "in ballet," at least she knew she was working with syntax, diction, psychosexual history. There was the potential for sustained expression. Using MTV as a model for narrative technique, however, is just a quick and dirty grab at her subject.

But then, maybe Armitage doesn't care about Milken as much as she says she does, and she set out to make junk theater, the performance version of junk bonds. Or maybe she hadn't noticed that Robert Wilson's best works have momentous scores to help them cohere, that Pina Bausch brings a spectacular focus to her weary intellectual striptease. The only zing of concentration in *The Predators' Ball* came from a black rapper who appeared in the piece. The collected energy he brought to the stage was like a wake-up call—he had a language. A narrow, low-ceilinged language, yes, but in this setting its simple authority and dexterity were greater than all the angles Armitage played. Post-dream, post-Balanchine, post-text, post . . . next? At BAM the post-narrative world is as weightless as ever.

December 1996

Misha: Impossible

The picture that sized up Mikhail Baryshnikov for his new audience in the West was an Avedon shot that ran in *Vogue* in October 1974, four months after the dancer defected. He flew straight up from the page, arms outstretched, chest bare, sky behind him—huge. He flew out of the lap of *Vogue* and into light. The move could have been the trick of a diver or a gymnast, but the body was pure ballet: that immaculate musculature, that privilege in space, those toes. Baryshnikov had chubby cheeks, which was a shock, and big, round, sad silent-movie eyes, a blue that sighed the word *persecution*. And it turned out he was small, about 5 feet 6 inches. So his round cheeks and round muscles and round-as-a-compass pirouettes and *tours en l'air* made him seem cherubic, a kind of opulent ballet angel. We knew he came from the Kirov, but with his blazing perfection he could just as easily have dropped from the sky, son of the sun. I remember tearing that photo out of *Vogue* and tacking it to the butter-yellow wall of my college dorm room.

The word *Apollonian* was soon tacked to Baryshnikov. In Gennady Smakov's book *The Great Russian Dancers*, you find him in the chapter titled "Dancers Without Category," an honor he shares with Vaslav Nijinsky and Rudolf Nureyev. All three came from the Kirov, all three popped the world's perception of the male dancer. But the first two were hotbloods who inspired writers to enraptured animal metaphors—big cats, golden slaves, jungle lust. As exotically and marketably Russian as Baryshnikov was, he did not channel Dionysus. He was more like the love child of pantherine, dance-or-die Nureyev and ice-cap cool, super-correct Erik Bruhn, dance gods of the sixties who had a romantic fascination with each other's techniques (and also a very brief fling). Misha was intense and aloof, charismatic and mega-correct, hot *and* cold. Though he was never dance-or-die like Rudi, when Baryshnikov was into his work it was all systems go, classical dancing on a par with Vladimir Nabokov on a literary riff: plush, precise, the pedant in a paradise of plosives. It was articulation pressing the boundaries of the language, self-consciousness at critical mass (eternity just beyond the sound barrier). Misha was a man, not a panther. That was the turn-on. His sensuality lay in his phenomenal formal purity. He was objectivity imploding, conservatism climaxing. Which is why he made such a match with choreographer Twyla Tharp, one of those feminists who only really respects men: They played mind games with the classical syntax.

In his dancing with American Ballet Theatre, Baryshnikov was always physically rapt, but over time his heart was missing. His Albrecht in *Giselle* became more false not less, as if Misha couldn't believe in the ballet anymore. The boil of his *brisés* in Act Two, a diagonal that always stunned the audience, they boiled harder, as if to heat up the performance. Eventually, Baryshnikov stopped dancing the prince roles. And that ravishing fifth position of his—legs crossed in an airtight X, thighs and calves having the tempered curves of Brancusi's *Bird in Space*—actually seemed less ballet's intimation of infinity than a place closed in, alone, a confessional molded to his use. It's funny, I can drum up memories of Baryshnikov dancing, but what floats up on its own is his face. I remember him looking out from his classical technique as if trapped in it.

Baryshnikov left ballet when he left his post as artistic director of ABT in 1989. He'd had it with the board, the development department, the whole arts-marketing circus. And he'd had it with the New York critics, who pooh-poohed his expensive production of *Swan Lake* and questioned his leadership of the company in ways they'd never questioned his dancing. American Ballet Theatre lost an imperfect, inspiring director and has been improvising ever since. And Baryshnikov? He defected again, this time quietly. In 1990, with Mark Morris, he founded a small modern dance company called the White Oak Dance Project.

But can he be a modern dancer? Last fall Baryshnikov made a guest appearance with the Tricia Brown Company at BAM's Next Wave Festival. Together, they danced her solo *If You Couldn't See Me*. It was a startling embodiment of the old adage, "You can take the boy out of fifth position but you can't take fifth position out of the boy." There was Brown, in her pigeon-toed, plain-Jane, haywire style—indecision in action—and there was Baryshnikov, doing the same steps at the same time ten feet away, making them look like commandments cut in travertine, neat, deep, decisive. The antithesis of the Brown style, he pulled the eye away from Brown and made the dance *his* solo (she became periphery). Such favoritism wasn't supposed to happen, but you can't blame the brain waves for seeking order.

He does look different these days. A picture of Baryshnikov by Fergus Greer ran in *The New Yorker* a week before White Oak's BAM engagement. The face that used to be so round is now lean, that used to be all cheek is now all forehead (the Luke Skywalker hair has been shorn). Baryshnikov's expression is stern, even severe, gravity pulling at his chin. And the shot itself puts him in a tight frame in which he doesn't fully fit and yet attempts to do a dance (actually, an awkward, right-angle hand position from Merce Cunningham's *Septet*). This photo sums up Baryshnikov's situation in the White Oak Dance Project. That ballet space and sky is long gone.

The name *White Oak* comes from a Florida-Georgia plantation owned by the Gilman Paper Company, whose chairman, Howard Gilman, has put money into the project and given it a place to work. The name also proposes a kind of parallel stature: Baryshnikov has left the pillars of classicism for the equally wise and pure Earth Mother oaks of modern dance. Nevertheless, it's not a particularly coherent or categorical bunch of dances he's put together, and there seems to be no curatorial basis for what's included. White Oak reads like a personal collection of totems and taboos, a repertory that revolves around Baryshnikov, what he thinks he should try and what he doesn't want to do again (i.e., anything he did before). He's cultivating a garden of think pieces and abstinence. Or to put it another way, there's too much forehead and not enough cheek.

It's been a long time since I've seen such a dour assemblage of dances. Both programs contained the late Erick Hawkins's last dance, *Journey of a Poet*, a work made in 1994 as a solo for Baryshnikov, and expanded posthumously into an ensemble. Set to a swarming string quartet, Hawkins's creepy-crawly *plastique* moderne makes *Poet* seem a crawl through Kafka, an abstraction of Baryshnikov's late-eighties Broadway performance as the cockroach in *Metamorphosis. Poet* is baloney, and also cause for concern. Doesn't Baryshnikov see how bad it is?

Both programs also featured the engagement's premiere, *Remote*, a long and punishingly austere ensemble work by young choreographer Meg Stuart (with equally punishing string music by Eleanor Hovda). Warning bells went off when I read André Lepecki's program note, a two-hundred-word tone poem that described *Remote* as "a dance moving around the limits of dancing. Reversing time, cutting time, expanding it to its annihilation . . ." Luckily I had read the *New York Times* the previous Sunday, where Stuart explained that she was actually deconstructing a pirouette. And so *Remote* begins with dancers spaced out (both meanings), inching around in glacial slow motion, belaboring the head snap of a ballet "spot," succumbing to *Le Sacre* spasms, starting over and over again. Time expands.

As for annihilation—grainy, gray slide projections of lost highways, barbed wire, empty windows, and blurred crowds hit the cyclorama in narrow shafts, like St. Sebastian arrows in the social skin. That pirouette, if you hadn't already guessed, is symbolic. Pirouettes, like man, are self-involved and solipsistic, isolated and alienating. Pretty soon the pirouettes look not deconstructed so much as detonated. It's a stage full of victims, everybody tripping and lurching, blown up and homeless. Two dancers try to "only connect." Only they can't. Baryshnikov does a pretty good imitation of a bum who's needling the audience and nodding off. The dance ends with Jamie Bishton in a cone of dust motes, convulsed.

That Stuart sustains the first half of *Remote*, the pirouette part, with such tonal security is an accomplishment. The dance is also slickly performed. But Stuart's heavy, high-school message is clichéd and dated. And on the evidence of *Remote*, her choreographic

Landscape with Moving Figures

hand is echt eighties, her sense of the body in space something between Twyla Tharp's violent off-centeredness and Anna Teresa de Keersmaeker's repeating decimal expressionism. I'm not surprised that most of Stuart's work has been commissioned and performed in Europe. They eat urban angst for breakfast.

The two swing dances on the programs offered respite, though they too were lit low and dusty. Merce Cunningham's *Septet* is an early charmer, one of the last dances in which he choreographed hand in hand with the music, Satie's *Three Pieces in the Shape of a Pear*. Cunningham not only teases his title—the dance requires six dancers (Les Six?)—he teases the twenties of Satie and St. Denis, posing his dancers in archly arty "modern dance" tableaux, framing them in air quotes, in Satie's moments of studied stillness. With Baryshnikov at its center, you feel Marcel Marceau in the air, too, for Misha plays happily with Cunningham's mimelike emphasis. It's perhaps more than Cunningham would wish for, but endearing all the same.

Unspoken Territory, a 1995 solo by Dana Reitz for Baryshnikov, was the blessing of the engagement. It is performed in silence, with Baryshnikov costumed in a chiton, apricot-shaded and sheer—he seems a Grecian ghost. And in fact he begins the piece in relief, as if he'd danced right off the surface of an urn, the power of his profile still acting upon him. It is a stream-of-consciousness solo, a passage of unheard melodies. Jennifer Tipton's lighting is a succession of half-lit geometries—pyramids and trapezoids—beamed down from the fly space, pitched in from the wings, widening and narrowing. Baryshnikov travels along rims of light, bobs in jars of shadow, strikes majestic poses in silhouette. He turns himself to stone, a centurian's horse, wakes suddenly to his own image and fingers his face like Narcissus. Free association gives way to refrain. In a repeating sequence of two steps, a leap, and a landing, the rhythm of his feet on the floor is so powerfully certain that the sounds—scuff, scuff, silence, and a *plumph*—come to seem code for the secret self. That airborne absence is the closest Baryshnikov comes to touching his soul in this repertory.

Unfortunately, *Unspoken Territory* doesn't compensate for the pleasureless, lusterless whole, the lack of kinetic kick. It's hard not to feel there's something punitive in this project, hard not to hear Baryshnikov saying something like, You didn't appreciate me at ABT, didn't see how serious I really was. I may be reading this in, and it may be unfair, but at the very least, White Oak shows his taskmaster's taste for the dogmatic and the cold, how he takes seriousness way too seriously. Why such dark tones and gloomy lighting? Why must string quartets sound like crazed cicadas or Soviet experiments? Why no joy, and so few jumps? Baryshnikov's solos are so *à terre* you'd think he ordered the air off-limits. And yet in the instances when he performed a jeté (in *Septet*), a series of turning leaps (the Hawkins), you felt a sigh go through the audience . . . *it's him, he's dancing*.

Who is Baryshnikov in this company? Large and lordly on the ballet stage—and make no mistake, even standing still little Misha flooded the Metropolitan Opera House with his presence—Baryshnikov's chief challenge here is to blend in, stay small. In the sense that the stylistic requirements of these dances scale him down, make him human, he does blend. He dances with modesty and commitment and splendid articulation. But without classicism there's no critical mass, and without mass there's no Misha. It's tempting to view Baryshnikov, in his self-imposed downsizing, as a statement on the diminished state of ballet. I suspect he wouldn't fight that interpretation. But I don't think it's that simple. Baryshnikov has always had a withholding side. He used to give his audiences wonder upon wonder. Now he wants to make us work.

May 1997

Frederick Ashton's England

The biggest dance event of the 1997 spring season was the publication of a book, Julie Kavanagh's *Secret Muses: The Life of Frederick Ashton*. The whispering chorus of kudos began last fall, when a lucky few New Yorkers got advance copies out of England, where the book was first published. Everything about *Secret Muses* felt right. Kavanagh had herself been a dancer, so there was understanding. She'd had Ashton's trust (and intimate chat) far beyond the extent he was willing to trust (and intimately chat with) any other journalist. And she'd been patient—the book was ten years in its meticulous making. It didn't hurt that Kavanagh made no pretense for her book as critical biography. While there are many passages in which she discusses Ashton's ballets, offering perspectives that new biographical data have brought into view, she never gets revisionist or self-righteous, sure ways to trigger the competitive instincts of critics. A tour de force of warmth, wit, and love for its subject, Kavanagh's book is, in a word, Ashtonian.

The timing was right, too. For New York City balletomanes, watching with exhaustion and ennui as the spirit of George Balanchine wanes at the New York City Ballet, *Secret Muses* arrived as an absorbing break from our own ballet problem. Or rather, it was a chance to ponder somebody else's problem, in this case, the waning spirit of Frederick Ashton at the Royal Ballet. When—as if on cue—the Royal Ballet landed at the Metropolitan Opera House for two weeks in July, comparison was in the air. And not just because the Royal could boast only one true-blue ballerina, Darcey Bussell, a dancer the company sometimes shares with the New York City Ballet (guest ballerinas have become a norm at NYCB, where the top of the roster is perilously thin). And not just because the Royal brought Ashton's *La Valse*, a work from 1958 that one couldn't help measuring against Balanchine's *La Valse* of 1951.

It is hard to read of Ashton's life and achievement in *Secret Muses* (those muses, not so secret within the ballet world, tended to be male dancers) without feeling the invisible pressure and standard of George Balanchine just across the pond. Both Ashton and Balanchine were born in 1904. Both revered Marius Petipa, choreographer of the Russian Imperial Ballet, and claimed his *Sleeping Beauty* as a touchstone in life and art (Petipa died in 1910). Both men were the founding choreographers for definitive new ballet companies: Ashton, with director Ninette de Valois, was the root of the Sadler's Wells Ballet, which became the Royal Ballet; Balanchine, with Lincoln Kirstein, was the soul of the New York City Ballet. And both men died in the 1980s, each surname symbolic of a classical style of dancing that is now in jeopardy. Their ascents through the thirties, the forties, the fifties, fly side by side. If Ashton became a national hero in England sooner than Balanchine did in America, Balanchine ascended higher, died at the helm of his company, and never had to see where it would go without him. Not so lucky, Ashton was replaced by choreographer Kenneth MacMillan in 1970, and his spotty representation in Royal repertory during the eighties and nineties remains a blot on the company. (In New York, audiences have always hungered for Ashton, the only contemporary on Balanchine's poetic level. It was a glorious collection of Ashton ballets that lent the Joffrey Ballet its magic in the eighties.)

As for the differences between the two choreographers: Balanchine was Russian and heterosexual; Ashton, English and homosexual. Reviewing *Secret Muses* in *The New Yorker*, Arlene Croce writes, "The biggest difference between the two choreographers was the emphasis that Ashton gave to the female upper body and Balanchine to the lower. Balanchine thought that a woman's expressive power was mainly in her legs and pelvis, Ashton in her head, upper back, and shoulders." This difference, Croce deduces, "betrayed their sexual orientation." As much as I appreciate the neatness of Croce's hypothesis, it is absurdly reductive, like saying the resolution of themes in Schubert's *Unfinished* Symphony proves he's gay. Yes, Balanchine concentrated on lower-body power and expression, and yes, Ashton was often caught up in the halo of *épaulement*. This difference, however, seems to me less one of sexual orientation (both men were, after all, unabashed romantics, serially infatuated fools for love) than of differing footholds on classical dance, i.e., their training.

Ashton said this much himself in 1984, in a review of Bernard Taper's book *Balanchine*. He wrote, "Balanchine has had all the necessary environment and background for the making of the great choreographer that he is. Unlike myself, who had to make all my opportunities from the beginning, and fight my way against every kind of prejudice in order to be allowed to dance. . . . all the Russian fairies must have gathered at his christening to bestow on him all his great gifts." Balanchine was practically born to ballet, taken into the Imperial School at age nine, whereas Ashton, having at thirteen seen Anna Pavlova perform ("She injected me with her poison and from the end of that evening I wanted to dance"), had to wait until he was twenty to take his first lesson. As anyone who has ever studied ballet knows, legs and feet are hardest and must be learned young. You can finesse the arms, but you can never fake legs. Ballet legs are conceptually complex, their power born in the pelvic bowl, fired in the torque of turn-out, the energy flowing fast, free, yet exquisitely through hip, knee, and toe. Ashton didn't have ballet in his body the way Balanchine did, a consummation as metaphysical as it is muscular (a consummation Ashton devoutly wished). He compensated with imagination, with stylish port de bras, and with ballets that were often heavily scripted, their clever, edgy librettos written by Edith Sitwell and Gertrude Stein.

Indeed, Ashton's ballets are often quite pointed, full of elaborate punctuation and exclamation. While Balanchine, from the beginning, understood the pointe as a form of divination, a key into ether (in the first bars of *Serenade*, when the stage of seventeen women snap their toes open into first position, you feel as if the lock on eternity has sprung), an Ashton pointe was an end in itself, a still point of perfection (in Ashton's *Cinderella*, Act Two ends with a rich, Leonardo-esque web of stage perspectives, all lines and eyes aimed toward Cinderella's empty pink-satin pointe shoe, symbol of *la danse*). Balanchine knew ballet from the inside out. Ashton was working from the outside in, trying to fill that shoe.

Look to 1946, a breakthrough year for both choreographers—but what different breakthroughs. Balanchine created *The Four Temperaments*, a ballet to Hindemith that seemed to burst out of nowhere, unprecedented in Balanchine's canon and in all of ballet. It begins with a man and woman standing side by side like Adam and Eve. They present their pointed toes to the audience, then, in a spasm of knowledge, they flex them. Those fierce feet lead them into maelstroms, into a syntactical hall of mirrors, into modernism, pelvis following in thrusts and swoons and sidlings. The *4Ts* is a ballet of sandstorms, scientific weights and measures (even its abbreviation sounds like a mathematical formula). Its dancers are outside ballet's Eden, searching among the sphinxes.

Meanwhile, over in England, Ashton premiered *Symphonic Variations*, and then staged his heraldic *Sleeping Beauty*. These ballets did not dive into chaos, they were acts of conservation, containment. It helps to remember that America, where Balanchine was, had dropped the atomic bomb in 1945. England, meantime, was living with unexploded shells in London gardens. While Balanchine was splitting anatomical atoms, Ashton was writing his first great couplets with the kind of classical transparency he'd longed for. He was entering the enchanted circle. Those two versions of *La Valse* suggest this difference. Both men hear Ravel driving toward oblivion, both ballets are costumed in doomy chic. But Ashton refuses to break out of his ballroom. He gives us Ravel's "whirling crowd" in ravishing washes, while Balanchine pierces the darkness, plunges into horror.

In other words, in 1946 Balanchine was actively breaking rules and making his own—opening the hip, moving weight off the heel—while Ashton was only just attaining the rules, which he adored as only an outsider can. He loved the planes of classicism: the fixed directions of the body on stage (there are eight), the well-anchored fifth position, the very square attitude, the golden mean of the low arabesque. It is this continuing eye contact with classical proportion that imbues Ashton ballets with their delicate equilibrium, their secret moral imperative, as if ballet was worth dying for. "Choreography is my whole being, my whole life, my reason for living," Ashton told writer David Vaughan. Living for, dying for, it is the same thing. And so English. This is what Ashton's postwar ballets of 1946—*Symphonic Variations* and *The Sleeping Beauty*—so achingly express.

The Royal Ballet came to New York as part of the summer's Lincoln Center Festival, and presented a sort of bookends approach to English ballet. It opened with the late Sir Kenneth MacMillan's final full-length work, *The Prince of the Pagodas* (1989), proceeded to the first full-length classical ballet ever staged by a British choreographer, Ashton's *Cinderella* of 1948, and dropped in an all-Ravel evening of repertory: works by Ashton, MacMillan, and budding choreographer Christopher Wheeldon.

Cinderella was a revelation. A few years ago, a rash of *Cinderella*s hit town—feminist versions, Nureyev's Hollywood production, the film *Pretty Woman*—the usual attempts to make it relevant. Instinct sent me in search of Ashton, and I found a very old, black-and-white tape of the ballet with Ashton and Robert Helpmann as the stepsisters, and Margot Fonteyn as Cinderella. I've never forgotten the hopefulness of Ashton's shy sister, her long horse face and Sun King wig, the jiggly precision of her big-bosomed, pebble-sized steps. And the unadorned fantasy of Cinderella's solos, so true to human nature. Where other productions layer on the cuteness, undermining Cinderella's moments alone by casting dancers as her cat or broom-come-to-life or you name it, Ashton has her tie a rag to a real broom (the rag is the arms) and dance lovingly with it.

Ashton has taken the episodic, even abrupt, Prokofiev score and given it a sensation of glide, perhaps by answering its moody shifts with such sure theatricality. The scurrying, squabbling Abbott-and-Costello act of the stepsisters—a pair portrayed as grotesquely lewd or vicious in almost every other *Cinderella* I've seen—are here slapstick of a celestial order, all the more hilarious (and poignant) because we like them so much. Whenever Cinderella's theme steals into the score, the ballet moves forward on a current of calm and longing. "To keep in a three-act ballet such a tone," Edwin Denby wrote in his review of 1949, "to sustain it without affectation or banality, shows Ashton's power, and he shows this in doing it as simply as possible, by keeping the dancing sweet." Still, sweetness does not come at the expense of invention. Corps work in *Cinderella*—the Seasons, the Hours, the Stars—is quick and brilliant, so quick and light you don't register its intricacy until a second viewing.

In his book *Frederick Ashton and His Ballets*, David Vaughan notes that at the time of its premiere there were complaints about *Cinderella*'s finale, a pas de deux for the Prince and Cinderella that struck some as too short and not grand enough. Ashton explained that there wasn't music for a big pas de deux (as opposed to the Wedding pas in *The Sleeping Beauty*), and, in fact, one of the immense pleasures of Ashton's ballet is that finale, a lingering dance back among the castle columns, which seems to occur on borrowed time. The last moments see Cinderella lifted high above the Prince's head, leg in attitude, as he carries her up some stairs, slowly turning all the while. Beyond the stairs is an arch, and beyond the arch a midnight-blue sky against which Cinderella's airborne attitude—the position of Mercury—spirals. It's as if she is passing from message to messenger to medium. Ashton's *Cinderella* hadn't been presented in New York in over twenty years. To see it live for the first time, as late as July 1997, was to remember why I love ballet.

At intermission during the company's matinee performance of *Cinderella*, I joined a group of critics outside. They were silent—sunstruck I thought (it was a high, hot sun)—but it turned out that they were feeling as I was, struck speechless by this luminous ballet. I wondered aloud about Royal dancing under Ashton, which I had never seen. How different did today's dancers look in *Cinderella*? The verdict: There is far less chiaroscuro today. The Ashton instrument was multi-articulated—head, shoulders, waist, hips, feet—each properly placed and planed in relation to the rest, like one of those wooden artist's models made up of spools threaded with elastic. Add to that a regard for etiquette. The placement of Margot Fonteyn, Moira Shearer, and Antoinette Sibley, as viewed on videotape, has always made me think of teacups in saucers being offered to the queen—the torso is a fraction forward and up. Of course, it doesn't take much eye to see that the international style toward which all the world's ballet companies are tending (courtesy of the global village)—a fusion of Balanchine speed, Bolshoi bigness, Forsythe androgyny—is hostile to Ashton. The Ashton articulation, the Cecchetti ticktock that lies under its ring pillow aplomb, has been swept up and lost in the larger torrents of our time, in our freer, less finicky, and more phenomenal approach to technique.

You can see it happening in the work of Ashton's successor, Sir Kenneth MacMillan, who maintained the Ashton footwork and quirky *épaulement* (the gold coins of English classicism), yet deeply distrusted the romance, the illusions, and instead created historically sweeping works that were the doomed and decadent flip side of fairy tales: *Romeo and Juliet*, *Manon*, *Mayerling*, *Anastasia*. By the time MacMillan got to *The Prince of the Pagodas*, which he fashioned as homage to *The Sleeping Beauty*, he had no love left. This fairy tale is formless and faithless, Aurora in the rubble, trapped in an undanceable score by Benjamin Britten (it's a ballet that wants to be an experimental opera). *Pagodas* is at its best when most Ashtonian: in the pointillist, personalized solos for Darcey Bussell, meditations that knit her steep scale to sewing-sampler footwork.

Ashton was no stranger to the decadent or nihilistic undertone. His *Les Illuminations*, choreographed for the New York City Ballet in 1950, tells the story of randy Rimbaud through sly subversions of classical clichés (corps groupings straight out of *Swan Lake*, etc.). But Ashton's sensibility was essentially positive and pastoral and communal, in the vein of Jane Austen. "It was a sweet view," writes Austen of the countryside in *Emma*, "sweet to the eye and mind. English verdure, English culture, English comfort, seen under a sun bright without being oppressive." She could be writing about Ashton's ballets. That landscape, that light, that enduring surround—these are as true of the abstract *Symphonic Variations* as they are of the storybook *La Fille mal gardée*. Ashton, like Austen, projects a sense of spirited enclosure. As always in great choreography, such intonations can be traced to technical mechanisms.

Balanchine and Ashton embody opposing states of grace. In ballet language, you might call these states *effacé* (shaded or open) and *croisé* (crossed). These terms do not denote steps but how the body is angled on its axis and in relation to the audience. To oversimplify, *effacé* is more loosely fixed and unbound, the step more open to the audience; in *croisé*, the body is at an oblique angle, with one leg barring our view to the other, a sort of fence between audience and dancer. Balanchine's vision as a choreographer was toward large-scale legibility, an omniscient openness, a sense of repertory as cosmos. Steps presented in *effacé* may be shaded—and Balanchine was a master of glancing shadows—but they are also freer of limb, the hips less weighted, thus allowing more hyperbole into the step, more height and momentum, release and flow. *Croisé* is at the heart of Ashton, his cross-my-heart-and-hope-to-die dedication to ballet. *Croisé* pins the dancer to the stage, creating instant tension between the hips and the upper body. It is exquisitely precise and protected. And it is modest. *Croisé* is Ashton's poetic temperament, the pasture gate upon which his heroine muses, the Highbury hedge that secures the dancer within the dance. In his famous essay, "Emma and the Legend of Jane Austen," Lionel Trilling invokes Schiller to point up Austen's moral system, how her novels play into the genre of the idyll as Schiller defined it: a hope for harmony, equilibrium, "the calm that follows accomplishment." Trilling's insight is relevant to Ashton. Where Balanchine chased his ideals (and ideal woman) into opalescent atmospheres, Ashton created idylls—that state, in the words of Schiller, "to which civilization aspires."

The third choreographer represented during the Royal's Met engagement was Christopher Wheeldon, whose *Pavane pour une infante défunte* was on the all-Ravel program. Wheeldon's pedigree is interesting. It includes training at the Royal Ballet School, a brief stint with the Royal Ballet, and, since 1993, dancing with the New York City Ballet. In June, NYCB presented a new ballet by Wheeldon as part of its third Diamond Project, a mini-festival showcasing the work of young choreographers. Of the six premieres in the project, it was Wheeldon's *Slavonic Dances* that brimmed with promise, that looked as if its choreographer was working from the ground up, attempting to build a ballet with interior allusions, not riding empty and amorphous trends. The music was Dvořák, and Wheeldon had still photographs by Josef Sudek projected on the cyclorama, a hint of the haunted, old-world atmosphere he was trying to conjure.

His ballet was too complicated and unfocused, however, filled with big moments that didn't satisfy. So many choreographers mistakenly equate the outlandish stunt with an event, forgetting that the kind of events we remember in ballets are often small moments the choreographer makes room for, those shoots through space to sudden seeing. When Ashton's Cinderella, partnered by her prince, moves into an arabesque facing the back right corner of the stage and then turns her face over her shoulder to smile at the audience, it is crushingly inclusive and happy. When Balanchine's Clara Schumann (in *Robert Schumann's "Davidsbündlertänze"*) looks down to see her husband's hand on her hip and secures it there with her own hand as if feeling for a sword, she has shown us her love in a locket. Wheeldon's *Slavonic Dances* was both imaginative and uneventful, an odd mix.

Pavane pour une infante défunte, a pas de deux from 1996, is another story—powerful beyond its means, events blossoming one after the other. *Pavane* lives somewhere between Ashton and Balanchine. In Wheeldon's choreography for the man there is something of Balanchine's airy expansion, his watchful, waiting male. In Wheeldon's choreography for the woman, pure pulses of Ashton. She first appears to us posed like Sargent's Madame X, her torsioned stance a stay against intimacy. Her next move—bourrées across the stage—are instantly emotional. They emerge, escape, from that pose. A giant calla lily that is the only decor breathes overhead of death (the child of the title?). And this man, is he her lover, her brother? She runs from him, leaves the stage, but always returns for his support. *Pavane* is an enigma variation, a ballet of containment and flight, at once Edwardian and modern. It is the best new ballet I've seen in a long while: a pact between *croisé* and *effacé*.

October 1997

Computer Games

In 1940, Martha Graham choreographed *El Penitente* and cast her handsome heartthrob, Erick Hawkins, as the Penitent. The young Merce Cunningham was a Christ figure. That same year, Graham choreographed a dance about Emily Dickinson, *Letter to the World*, and cast Hawkins as the Dark Beloved. Cunningham was the poet's elfin wit. In 1944, Graham choreographed *Appalachian Spring* and cast Hawkins as the Bridegroom. Cunningham was a preacher.

Graham may have been concentrating hard on Hawkins, who was indeed her dark beloved and eventual, if skittish, bridegroom, but her take on Cunningham is the more piercing portrait. Christ figure, cool humorist, guru—all true. Cunningham would leave Graham's company in 1945, would head to Black Mountain College with John Cage, where, in a forty-days-forty-nights kind of immersion (actually about two years), they would create an aesthetic that was antithetical to Graham theatrics (and far more lighthearted), and would do nothing less than redefine purity in the theater, trading impulse for pulse, and feeling for seeing. Here at the end of the twentieth century, after more than forty years of dance-making, Cunningham is still a visionary. While the great Paul Taylor, in his rippling universe of leaping Manichean extremes, moral solstice and eclipse, plays God à la Dr. Jekyll, Cunningham plays Consciousness.

In other words, he plays. What Cunningham and Cage fixed on so early and threateningly was the notion that the toss of a coin, the roll of the dice, the reading of tea leaves or the *I Ching*, was as viable a way to organize a dance as any other. Chance was God. Chance was opportunity, the orange card in the board game—a chance to escape the monopoly of ingrained artistic strategies. The scholar Roger Copeland, in his book *Merce Cunningham: The Modernizing of Modern Dance*, puts it thus: "Cunningham remains skeptical about the role that 'natural' and unconscious impulses play in the creative process.... Indeed, Cunningham makes a point of resisting his own 'instinctive' preferences (which is to say: the preferences that *feel* natural)." He isn't into the power of id, or the auteur's omnipotence. In fact, in her 1991 biography of Martha Graham, Agnes de Mille recalls that Cunningham did not care for his role as the preacher in *Appalachian Spring*, and in the solo he himself choreographed "showed more anger than was needed." Was he already uncomfortable with the artist's Promethean reach, or too comfortable with it? (No one has ever accused Cunningham of being simple.)

And so the choreographic elements of a Cunningham dance (the order of pre-choreographed sections, the length of those sections, the number of dancers in sections, etc.) were decided upon by alien or arbitrary forces. Likewise, the composer and the designers did their work in the dark, without jam sessions on what it was all meant to express. Not until the first performance did the elements inhabit the same time and space, or the dancers hear the music (they knew the dance by counting) and wear the costumes. It was as if the dance had a mind of its own beyond Cunningham and his collaborators. Obviously, this creational void sitting at the back of each work made critics nervous. How do you review chance?

Forty years later, critics are still trying to answer that question. On the last day of Cunningham's week-long October engagement at the Brooklyn Academy of Music, part of this year's Next Wave Festival, a panel called "Writing About Merce" was convened. The problems discussed were easy to identify with, for writer and watcher alike. Take the absence of conventional music, aural structures that would cue you to where you are in a piece—this makes it difficult to remember steps, to fix them in a phrase. (It can also scare you into thinking the dance will never end.) And all those chance operations, they seem to wave away a committed analysis of a work. And if you do impose autobiography or allegory or imagery on a work, are you not betraying it? Yet during an intermission chat I had with Douglas

Dunn, one of Cunningham's first and most famous dancers, Dunn complained that critics never write about what the dances mean.

This anxiety about meaning is like an X factor at the core of Cunningham, an unknown in the mathematical formula (a sensation of higher math pervades both steps and sound, as so many of the scores consist of electronic oscillations and waves—E=merce^2). A dance from 1989 called *Cargo X* could be a little key to Cunningham. In it, a backstage ladder brought onstage figures first as a prop, a ladder. It then begins to assume the iconic stature of an obelisk, exerting a pull on the dancers. Finally, as the dancers lay flowers on its rungs, the ladder has become a monument or tombstone. Cunningham's "cargo" is bodies and time and change. In short, life and death. But Cunningham would never say so.

The most beautiful of the four new dances on Cunningham's two BAM programs was *Installations*, a work from 1996 that plays, even puns, with an equation Cunningham walked away from when he walked away from Graham: the idea of Art as Church, an institution that "installs" spirit. As we all know by now, art installations tend to be big, empty spaces, usually with an electronic buzz piped in, often with a video screen nearby. Cunningham's *Installations* has a decor by Elliot Caplan. Three banks of video screens (each made of four or six screens) are positioned asymmetrically around the stage; a graceful swath of curtain is the backdrop. Pieced together within each bank of screens is a looming, stone-gray video of a stone-still (but breathing) dancer. They're like refractions of the sculpted saints and angels you'd see in a cathedral, and they catch something of the height, the isolating scale and sentience of cathedrals. Caplan's lighting drapes the dance in Vatican gradations of rust, garnet, grape; and Trimpin's score, at first art-museum minimal, gathers and grows throaty like organ chords, but chords played by the church cat lounging on the keys. When, amid a stageful of shadowy groupings, light falls on the feet of two dancers, each left foot tensed in the same demi-pointe position, it's nothing less than an Adoration. Again, forget the preacher. *Installations* is like eyes wandering—a mind wandering—during the sermon.

The hot dance on the program was the world premiere *Scenario*, a must-see for the cutting-edge set because of its costumes by Rei

Kawakubo, founder of the fashion house Comme des Garçons. Kawakubo is that rarity, a truly avant-garde fashion designer. Disdainful of trends, her own as well as others', her mantra is "Starting from Zero"—she is constantly starting over or subverting the norm. For instance, she'll loosen a screw in the weaving machines to get imperfection, chance, back into mass-produced fabric. As for shape, her three-armed sweater was a semiotician's dream.

The much-awaited costumes for *Scenario* were versions of dresses Kawakubo showed a year ago in her spring 1996 collection, or, as some of the fashion press called it, the "Quasimodo" collection. Its signature silhouette was a body-hugging stretch dress with extra fabric bunched and pulled over tuberous humps and bumps in odd places (*Artforum* went crazy for it). Kawakubo said she was exploring human shape, testing and freshening the eye. But, she continued, if you slipped the down-filled pads out of their fabric envelopes you were left with a perfectly conventional stretch dress. The costumes the Cunningham dancers wore were dresses made in blue-and-white stripes or sea-foam gingham, followed by a group dressed in black, then one in irradiated tomato. The shapes were Disney animation—as if someone had loosened a screw in *that* machine—and the dancers looked like errant toadstools, or had Mighty Mouse chests and Popeye muscles, even Saturn rings around midriffs. Kawakubo's set was a bare, white stage with fluorescent lighting, a sort of ground zero.

The costumes stole the show. The colorful first section suggested a tropical utopia, an undiscovered island of dancing mutants. When the dancers came out in their black Kawakubos, I thought of French poodles groomed for show; Victorian widows, their bustles askew; the precarious black hair buns of geishas. I had not considered just how ubiquitous humps and bumps are in fashion history, how natural to the landscape of artifice. Nor had I ever seen the Cunningham dancers look glamorous in quite this way, in a fashion context. The women's strong, slim, lower legs were suddenly gorgeous, feminine legs. Eroticized. Gams.

But, O brightening glance, How can we know the dancer from the costume? *Scenario* was difficult to see, literally, like watching a screen in which the horizontal is out of whack with the vertical ("Do not attempt to adjust your television set . . ."). It was as if each dancer was moving within a sci-fi blur. Sit back and squint, and the stage picture was charming and bright, if untranslatable. Lean in and the dance was a bunch of arms and legs poking out of pillows. What was clear is that we have powerful expectations regarding Cunningham dancers. We not only want to see their bodies, we need to. The articulation of the Cunningham midsection (inner thigh, hip, waist, ribs, clavicle)—so crisp, specific, sensitive, and solid—is the quick of Cunningham, the seat of his Sensurround perception. In *Scenario*, he wasn't all there.

The same could be said for all four of the new dances (the two other New York premieres were *Rondo*, which had a motif of "watching," and *Windows*, a rather ominous, inscrutable work with the color scheme of wet cement). Despite their various scores, palettes, and motifs, all four works were distant. All four were busy. Even *Installations*, so quietly lovely, was more a triumph of its parts. None of these works had that sudden drop into intimacy that can make Cunningham seem the most wondrously sensual, the most listening of choreographers (the illumination of two feet in *Installations* was as intimate as it got). None had that unpredictable pull, almost barometric, into a pocket of concentration. This lack was brought into high relief by the *BAMevent*s that were also on the program. Pieces of older dances elided together to make a new dance just for that evening, the *BAMevent*s included sections of dances from the 1950s through the 1980s. The focused muscularity, the sheer sense of involvement in these snippets, presented quite a contrast. One felt the difference dimensionally, in the palpable zones of space around dancers, and theatrically, in the precision-burn speed, in a leg monumentally upheld—leg as will. One also realized, with a bit of a jolt, that there were no memorable pas de deux in any of the new dances. The *BAMevent* duet from *Un jour ou deux* of 1973—great chaste spirals and stillnesses—begged the question and left one longing for more.

The fact that John Cage died in 1992 may or may not have some bearing on the missing duets in Cunningham's latest works. The fact that Cunningham is now using Lifeforms, a computer program for choreographers, to create his dances and then to activate them (instead of dice or the *I Ching*) seems significant. Maybe you *can* review chance.

The distracted, disembodied quality of the four new dances certainly corresponds to the distracted, disembodied quality you get from pictures on computer screens. The carriage of the arms, so exact in Cunningham, so classically placed and yet quirky, brainy, was inexact and rather lost in the atmosphere. A fellow critic and avid Merce watcher was extremely bothered by those arms, and suggested that port de bras on the computer screen may be correspondingly inexact, a problem compounded by Cunningham's not making the dances on his own body anymore.

We have watched Cunningham, who is now seventy-eight, age within his dances, and it has been a fascinating, funny, and sometimes unsettling experience. He has never tried to do physically what he cannot, the way Rudolf Nureyev used to (Nureyev, who relished the role of Preacher in Graham's *Appalachian Spring*). He has used his older self choreographically, to make comments—humorous, sarcastic, sage, sad—on his position as aging master among young bodies. But watching Cunningham's physicality pass out of his dance-making, taking with it that tough muscular intelligence, that acute attunement to pitches beyond the rest of us, is adjustment of another order. Cunningham, however, would probably say it's all in the game.

December 1997

Balanchine's Castle

This winter, *Jewels* reappeared in New York City Ballet repertory the way it does every few years, like a mirage of overwhelming majesty, a floating castle set amid fairy forests and ancient ice caps, a castle guarding its secrets. The night before the first performance, NYCB held a seminar on *Jewels* for its Guild members. Dancers from the ballet's premiere on April 13, 1967—Conrad Ludlow, Suki Schorer, and Edward Villella—were onstage to speak about that night, those steps, the rehearsals, and, of course, the ballet's choreographer, George Balanchine. The moderator, *Ballet Review* editor Francis Mason, began by explaining that Balanchine had a PR angle when he conceived *Jewels*: he thought Van Cleef & Arpels might foot the bill (lo, City Ballet got not a sou). It was also to be just one ballet, but when Balanchine began working, his idea grew. Soon there were two ballets, then three. In rehearsal, the work was referred to as "Jewels," but on the night of the premiere it went untitled because management was still waffling over what to call this strange evening. The three sections, however, were called "Emeralds," "Rubies," and "Diamonds."

The rehearsal title won out, and *Jewels* became famous as the "first three-act plotless ballet." Its sheer size was dazzling. As Ludlow explained at the seminar, "We were in transition still from City Center [to the New York State Theater at Lincoln Center] and I think that was one of the purposes of the ballet, part of the concept—the gigantic scale." Balanchine wanted to show that his dance and his dancers could fill this larger stage.

"There was a kind of pandemonium in the theater that night," said Suki Schorer, recalling that it wasn't until the premiere that the dancers knew they were taking part in a masterpiece. In *Thirty Years/The New York City Ballet*, Lincoln Kirstein writes, "*Jewels* has been an unequivocal and rapturous 'success' since its introduction, the very title sounds expensive before a step is seen." Rich is how *Jewels* really looks, and not so much in terms of money (the sets are minimal—parures of gemstones pasted on a bare backdrop). *Jewels* is immediately sensuous, saturated, a pleasure-dome decreed. Its crystal and glycerine surface is magic, but inside you begin to sense shadows, murmurs, and the undertow.

Indeed, the audience at the Guild Seminar seemed to be in a state of "I know, but I don't know what I know," for question after question was put to the dancers, each one ignoring the fact of *Jewels*'s plotlessness. Did Balanchine explain what was happening in *Jewels*? Did he tell you what it meant or was about? ("Rubies," Villella was told by Mr. B, was "about twenty minutes.") Did he discuss your character, your role? No, no, and no, came the answers. The castle was still guarding its secrets.

Jewels doesn't demand that you dissect it. It can be enjoyed as pure spectacle, beginning with the colors. The lighting design of Ronald Bates and the costumes of Madame Karinska work in brilliant complicity. Bates makes palpable poetic weather of his lighting, which Karinska's costumes either sink into ("Emeralds") or bounce out of ("Rubies") or refract ("Diamonds"). And so the French opaline greens that soften and blur the edges of "Emeralds" create a plush and pillowy space, a netherworld love nest. The sharp red of "Rubies" practically vibrates against a cindery light; it's a red with black in it, royal and radical at once. And the snow-crystal radiance of "Diamonds" is underlit with a blue as pale as a vein in a slim white wrist.

Karinska's costumes are knockouts. The tutus vary—long and misted in "Emeralds," hip-short and heraldic in "Rubies," stiff sprays in "Diamonds"—but all the bodices, whether green, red, or white, are glittering armatures, intricately seamed and encrusted with jewels, part Tennyson, part Dior. These bodices are fascinating. That reverse décolleté, a passementerie of jewels curving *under* each breast like baroque scrollwork, leaves the bosom naked (actually, sheathed in nude fabric). It's an odd and erotic eye-catcher, suggesting maidens framed in high windows, awaiting the troubadour's song. That song is different in each section, and thus *Jewels*'s faceting begins.

Much has been written about the three parts or panels of *Jewels*, and they can be differentiated with ease. "Emeralds" is French, set to romantic Fauré, dreamy and somnambulistic. "Rubies" is American, neoclassical Stravinsky, nervy and voracious. "Diamonds" is Imperial Russia, palatial Tchaikovsky, tender and at times ecstatically elegiac. You can keep *Jewels* in these compartments, and read it as a lavishly illustrated monograph on Balanchine's lifelong preoccupations, circa 1967: his experimentation with national styles of classical dancing, his exploration of his own aesthetic affinities—with Paris and Petipa, with Stravinsky and Tchaikovsky. You can even pop out a panel and perform it solo, as has been done with "Rubies" all around the world. But the wholeness of *Jewels* is also the power and glory of *Jewels*.

The score for "Emeralds" was pieced together by Balanchine from incidental music that Gabriel Fauré composed for two plays: Maurice Maeterlinck's *Pelléas et Mélisande* (1898) and a Shakespeare adaptation called *Shylock* (1889). It combines impressionist washes of sound, perfumed and yearning, with simple woodcut melodies that seem sprung from medieval lore. "Emeralds" finds Balanchine deep in the poetic realm of Coleridge and Keats—it's an enchanted forest filled with Darke Ladies—and within the compositional genre of hunt and vision scenes (*Swan Lake*, *The Sleeping Beauty*). It is a work of trance and transparency. You feel you can reach through the green of "Emeralds" and grasp nothing.

What explains this disconnection? To begin with, the pyramidal dance structures of "Emeralds"—its solos, duets, pas de trois, and ensembles—suggest a fairy court on the order of *A Midsummer Night's Dream*, and yet not one but two women are at the top: a first ballerina and, a faint shade beneath her, a second. The Paris Opéra–trained Violette Verdy originated the first role, and put her stamp on a solo that is like no other solo in Balanchine ballet. Intimate, bright, it's an aria of upper-body animation, hands, arms, and shoulders preening, self-regarding, scintillating—a Jewel Song. This ballerina wraps herself and her thoughts in pure port de bras (a Verdy specialty). She seems lost in some fantasy—or found—we do not know. The second ballerina also has a solo, but she is more famous for the "walking duet," a measured, measureless passage—on pointe—along a winding path in which she is supported by a man of whom she is unaware.

Verdy's solo is, in cinematic lingo, the ballet's establishing shot, for with this solo *Jewels* fixes on a pervasive Balanchine preoccupation—the unknowable woman. The second ballerina seconds it. The inequality of these two roles may be that the first is awake and the second asleep. Together, the two add up to a single ambivalence, a sensibility torn or in flux, like Titania in her two states (self-possessed, then spellbound by Oberon), or those twins in confusion, Hermia and Helena ("I have found Demetrius like a jewel/Mine own, and not mine own"). "Emeralds" ends with three men down on one knee like knights who have dismounted, their eyes sweeping the path for signs of her, the troubled ideal.

In "Rubies" the men have remounted—they're chess knights (and pawns)—and the girls are fillies, tomboys, pinups, Broadway gypsies, Gypsy Rose Lees, the whole high-kicking, gear-stripping gamut of leggy American allure. Stravinsky's percussive score, Capriccio for Piano and Orchestra, is syncopated like rush hour, then cocktails: you hear the subway rumbling underneath, feel neon Broadway and New York noir take over. In response to the "Rubies" = America equation, Balanchine has said, "I did not have that in mind at all." Nevertheless, the first glittering glimpse of "Rubies"—its cast holding hands upstage in a paper-doll arc, poised on pointe—never fails to draw a gasp of appreciation from the audience. It's a city skyline at night, the Big Apple ablaze.

It is in "Rubies" that you clearly see Balanchine using his jeweler's tools, concentrating on the angled body positions of classical dance—*écarté, effacé, croisé*—and throwing in *épaulé*, an upper-body arrangement that pulls the arms and torso in prismatic opposition to the lower body, creating a kind of dynamic duality, directional energies at cross purposes. All this was in "Emeralds," but subliminal, cloaked in haze and dew. "Rubies," so overtly athletic, is more pointed. Substitute leotards for those rich red Karinskas with their clacking plackets, and "Rubies" could take its place in Balanchine's black-and-white wing, next to the quantum physics of *The Four Temperaments* and *Agon*.

As in "Emeralds," there are two female leads in "Rubies," but this time one is a true principal, the other a soloist. The lead was originated by tiny Patricia McBride, the second by bigger Patricia Neary. "Rubies" belongs to McBride, but where she seems to be cozily throned in the pas de deux, that sirenlike second girl runs roughshod through the ballet, hitting cheesecake poses that drive the male corps mad. In one graphic sequence four men dive at her in succession, each grabbing a wrist or an ankle. They proceed to manipulate her into split *penchées* and leg extensions, again along the grammatical cuts of *effacé* and *écarté*. Mantrap or manhandled? This role is always cast with a tall girl. Her MO is seduction, and she is the "Rubies" theme writ large.

For smack at the center of "Rubies" is an encounter sui generis, a Genesis—the pas de deux originated by McBride and Edward Villella—and smack at the end of that is a tree. Not literally, but the pas de deux finishes with McBride standing downstage, her arms splayed like branches, Villella snug behind her and climbing around. In a nursery rhyme of intertwining limbs, Villella finally opens out a hand and McBride drops something invisible into his palm. It's that other apple, "Rubies" red.

The brilliance of McBride was that with her sinuous, spiky style she turned original sin into a one-woman show: in "Rubies" she's Eve *and* the serpent, the apple *and* the tree. Balanchine leads us to man's first story of seduction with a more recent story straight out of the ballet canon, though again McBride is the only ballerina who's truly shown it to us. The sensation of black one feels in the red of "Rubies" is none other than Odile, the black swan from *Swan Lake*, the imposter-swan who seduces the prince away from gentle white swan Odette, and destroys his life. There is a diagonal in "Rubies" straight out of the Black Swan pas de deux, as well as other Odile-isms—her distorted and dominating attitudes, her relentless pull on the man. McBride danced this pas de deux with come-hither casualness, a faux-swan insinuation and feline triumph. In "Rubies," Balanchine sees Woman as forbidden fruit, eternal Eve, downfall.

"Diamonds" has been called an "Odette fantasy," and as a friend recently observed, it feels like the fifth act—a wish fulfillment—of four-act *Swan Lake*. Actually, Tchaikovsky's Symphony no. 3, from which the music is taken, was composed in the summer of 1875, just months before Tchaikovsky began work on *Swan Lake*. There are links between the two scores in key and orchestration, almost as if Tchaikovsky was tuning up for *Swan Lake*, testing the waters (still cold), and feeling his way into the forest. Certainly Balanchine hears it this way. The pas de deux in "Diamonds" refracts imagery from the pas in *Swan Lake*'s Act Two: the vow of love, Odette's arrowy path (so like the winding path in "Emeralds"). In this act of *Jewels*, there is only one ballerina—Suzanne Farrell. She is aware of her isolation and the windswept forces around her.

Farrell was Balanchine's growing obsession throughout the 1960s, and when he choreographed *Jewels* the obsession was in full bloom. In a *New Yorker* essay on *Jewels* published in 1983, Arlene Croce writes, "If I had to guess how the piece was made, I'd say that Balanchine worked backward from the pas de deux of 'Diamonds'. . ." This is an assessment of Farrell's power as creative muse. Croce also describes how in "Diamonds," mixed in with the Odette iconography, there are pawing steps and forward extensions that allude to the unicorn in the Cluny tapestries. Croce's view is supported by Farrell, who writes in her autobiography of 1991, *Holding On to the Air*, of how Balanchine took her to the Musée de Cluny to see The Lady and the Unicorn tapestries. Of the sixth tapestry she writes: "He loved the title *A Mon Seul Désir* ["To My Only Desire"] and said he wanted to make a ballet for me about the story of the unicorn." It seems safe to say that "Diamonds" is that ballet, or rather, that *Jewels* is, that it was the white glow of the unicorn that Balanchine chased into the forest, only to find himself in a thicket of haunting and hunted creatures. Claude Debussy began at the end when he composed, with permission from Maeterlinck, the opera *Pelléas et Mélisande*. The first thing he wrote was the climactic Act Four love duet, as if to make for himself a white light at the end of the tunnel—which he needed because the forests of *Pelléas et Mélisande* are so thick and dark that "there are places where you never see the sun." What are these forests but the human psyche? And what is light but love? And who is Mélisande?

"Only the most beautiful emeralds contain that miracle of elusive blue," wrote Colette in *Gigi*. It is through elusive blue we must travel if we are to grasp *Jewels*, through Fauré and Debussy and Maeterlinck to the deep-sea mystery of Mélisande, the ingenue-soprano who has kept opera lovers guessing for almost a century. She is the central question of Maeterlinck's play, for she herself will give no answers. We, along with Golaud, the older man who marries her, know only where he found her. Maeterlinck's stage direction reads: *"A forest. Mélisande discovered at the brink of a spring."* It could be Balanchine's stage direction for "Emeralds." Mélisande is lost and weeping, has dropped the crown she was wearing into the spring, and will later drop her wedding ring there as well (a Freudian slip of the fingers). Pelléas is Golaud's younger half-brother, and he has instant affinity with Mélisande, which becomes love and leads to his death at the hand of Golaud. Where Pelléas believes in "the truth, the truth, the truth," Mélisande offers evasion, as if unversed in human rules. She nurses a secret sorrow, and is allied with water, fountains, the sea.

What—not who—is Mélisande, may be the better question. There are those who believe she is one of the water sprites immortalized (and they are immortal, unless they mix with humans) in Friedrich, Baron de la Motte Fouqué's story *Undine* (1811). Also, the name Mélisande is very like Mélusine, the undine of a famous French fairy tale. (Mélusine marries a human on the terms that he must never interrupt her privacy. Breaking the terms, he enters her chamber and finds her transformed, playing in a pool. She leaves him.) And in Debussy's *Pelléas et Mélisande*, a work of ravishing irresolution begun in 1893 and premiered in 1902, the closest the composer comes to a true aria occurs when Mélisande lets her otherworldly hair fall from a window. Mermaids are known for two things—their long hair and their song.

Although "Emeralds" has been likened to a tapestry, to chivalric France, to green earth, it has always been described with liquid images. Verdy commented on its "underwater quality," and Kirstein described it as a "submarine summer-green garden." In his book *George Balanchine*, Richard Buckle reports that in 1958 Balanchine had discovered the music of Fauré and imagined a "tipped ballroom" behind a scrim with "a projection of the sea . . . which pulsates." It not only makes musical-textual sense that the first ballerina in "Emeralds" is an undine, it also makes sense choreographically. In Verdy's solo, it is easy to see a woman modeling bracelets and tiaras, though when asked if Balanchine ever mentioned such jewelry, Verdy answered, "No. No bracelets." Might we not as easily see Undine or Mélusine splashing in her imaginative element, wearing water droplets like gems? In fact, it was only during this season's round of *Jewels* that those Karinska costumes—so charming, so puzzling—struck me with new depth. That bare bosom, accentuated by gem work, and those bodices so tightly seamed and sheathed beneath, recreate the naked flash and surge of mermaids.

"Rubies" is more Lorelei Lee than Undine, the golddigger with no regrets (rubies are a girl's best friend). But in "Diamonds" the blue-green waters of "Emeralds" turn to frost and ice. Tchaikovsky's hunting horns seem to answer the far-off horn calls in "Emeralds." Furthermore, Balanchine knew that the watery theme of *Swan Lake*'s Act Two—the lakeside pas de deux—was not original to *Swan Lake*. Tchaikovsky recycled it from an earlier, failed opera, *Undina*. Balanchine has given Farrell some swan queen flutterings, yet she also reiterates the liquid port de bras of Verdy's solo, with a heightened, perhaps frightened, emphasis. Where Verdy drew delight from her invisible spring center stage, Farrell draws strength and scale.

Move in close and *Jewels* acts more like a solitaire under a spotlight, a single gem glinting a spectrum of hue and allusion. *Jewels* is knee deep in French Symbolists, Mallarmé as much as Maeterlinck. Listen closely to Fauré, and you hear Debussy's tumescent woodwinds, Mallarmé's faun stretching in the leaves, wondering "Loved I a dream?" *Jewels* takes up the tensions of the Symbolists, who took up symbols of the Romantics before them—their use of the half-human to understand the human, their sense of the dislocation between possession and privacy, infatuation and freedom. *Jewels* is a vision touched with myths of transformation, with the conflicting impulses of escape and rescue. That the mermaid swims through all channels of *Jewels* is yet another flash of recognition: mermaids have always symbolized the free flow of the mind, the sea of the subconscious. The questions whispered in these waters and woods are the stuff of Balanchine's dreams, and they are unanswerable: To what extent can you possess a woman, a wife, a ballerina? To what extent can you own your only desire without killing it?

There is an alternate view to Mélisande's identity, and its meanings move deep and dark under *Jewels*. This analysis also comes by way of the opera. If Mélisande has dropped her crown into the spring, the obvious next question is, who gave her the crown? She says, "It is the crown he gave me. . . . I will have no more of it! I had rather die." The scholar Henri Barraud identifies Mélisande as one of Bluebeard's ex-wives escaped from his castle. Or perhaps she is a wife to be. One of Charles Perrault's more rigid and unforgiving stories (it's hard to call it a fairy tale), *Bluebeard's Castle* connects with *Pelléas et Mélisande* in its atmosphere of hot and cold unknowns, its Symbolist portents ripe with erotic suggestion. Another link is Maeterlinck himself. He wrote a version of the tale called *Ariane et Barbe-Bleue*, and he named one of the wives Mélisande.

In brief, *Bluebeard's Castle* is the story of old Bluebeard's young bride, who, in order to know him better, asks for keys to the seven locked doors in his castle. He gives her all the keys, but as a test of fidelity forbids her opening the seventh door. In some versions of *Bluebeard's Castle*—Béla Bartok's opera of 1918, for instance—the keys are given with no stipulations, only foreboding. In eerie empathy, Bartok's staging accompanied the opening of each door with a wash of color—*Jewels*-like lighting effects in red, blue-green, gold, and bright white. Beyond the doors are rooms, each room a facet of Bluebeard's wealth. We see one by one the torture chamber, the armory, the house of jewels, the garden, Bluebeard's lands, a Lake of Tears. Finally, from the seventh room, three ex-wives emerge, the loves of Bluebeard's dawn, noon, and evening. This new wife must take her place behind the seventh door as the wife of Bluebeard's nights.

Violette Verdy once coached Suki Schorer in her role in "Emeralds" and passed on the story she'd invented for herself. "It happens in a bedroom," Verdy insisted. Schorer, imagining a glorious Parisian apartment, repeated this interpretation to Balanchine, who replied, "No it doesn't." But Verdy's instincts ring true. *Jewels* does feel like a castle full of rooms, doors opening onto air. Without imposing Bluebeard too rigidly on Balanchine, you *can* see the kingdom's gardens and woodlands in "Emeralds." As for the torture chamber and armory, that would be blood-red "Rubies." At the seminar, Villella made no bones about the fact that his role in "Rubies" was a "gut cruncher," aerobically brutal. He asked Balanchine to change a long stretch that left him gasping for breath, and got one hardly helpful rest in the wings. And I go back to that moment in which the tall girl is manacled by four men, then drawn and quartered.

"Diamonds" is the sixth room, the Lake of Tears, for, as we know from the Act Two mime of *Swan Lake*, Odette resides in the lake made of her mother's tears. And "Diamonds" is the seventh room, too. Like Bluebeard, Balanchine had wives throughout his life. In 1967, when Balanchine was sixty-three, there were three ex-wives alive (plus one common-law ex, Alexandra Danilova); he was currently married to his fourth wife, Tanaquil Le Clercq; and was in love with the woman he wanted to be the fifth, the twenty-one-year-old Farrell. She was his Hope Diamond, the ballerina in *Jewels* who doesn't share the stage with a second because she was all women, all enchantments—unicorn, swan, undine—in one.

When Balanchine choreographed *Jewels*, he did not know Farrell would refuse him. They were still in the flush of their affinity, and the finale he put on "Diamonds"—not the suicide-apotheosis of *Swan Lake*, but a wedding coronation—reflects his hope for a happy ending. In her autobiography, Farrell tells of how she and Mr. B. went to Van Cleef & Arpels, and, "while cameras clicked away, George and M. Arpels threw priceless jewelry at me. They even took the crowns of Empress Josephine and the Czarina out of the vault and put them on my head. We were like children locked in a candy store." Or in the third room, the house of jewels.

Farrell didn't wish to stay locked in. Balanchine's ardor grew; he wanted to have and to hold, and in 1969, in an act of escape, Farrell married a dancer her own age, Paul Mejia. The couple was banished.

Filling the ballerina roles of *Jewels* once the first ladies left them has always been a company challenge, though these days it can feel more like a confrontation. The bigness of *Jewels* requires clarity and an air-cushion of commitment around that clarity. The romance of *Jewels* requires delicacy. Yet how small so many performances feel today.

Unlike McBride in "Rubies" and Farrell (who returned to the company in 1975) in "Diamonds," both dancing their roles well into the 1980s, Verdy left NYCB and "Emeralds" in the seventies. The most crucial ballet in *Jewels* because it is the one that casts the spell, "Emeralds" today is a scent without complexity, a profound evocation reduced to prettiness. It has been this way for a long time, and people have been complaining ever since Verdy left, though I've never forgotten Stephanie Saland in the role, smoky and remote. Neither Miranda Weese nor Kathleen Tracey was up to her level of imaginative interest, let alone Verdy's, though I had great expectations for Weese, who has been quietly sublime in some of the more stylistically distilled Balanchine roles—in the first movement of *Symphony in C*, for example, and the first movement of *Brahms-Schoenberg Quartet*—and who is the only young NYCB principal with upper-body sophistication.

Weese in "Rubies" was another story. While Margaret Tracey had great glitter, she tired visibly, showing chinks. Wendy Whelan had wit and snap, yet there was no sense of seduction, or, as critic Robert Greskovic put it, "no silk." Weese, however, put silky and sinful together, adding her own prancing élan. The longer she was onstage, the stronger and more tonally secure she got—and she took the audience with her. I've never seen a bare back used to such effect in this ballet. It somehow magnified her serenely correct carriage, which in turn called attention to her reserves of stillness, a facet of true musicality and something very rare in ballet today (though it didn't used to be rare). In start-and-stop "Rubies," Weese showed what a decisive, dramatic impact a full stop can have. In the three *Jewels* I saw, "Rubies" was the ballet that caught the audience—its energies are cracklingly coherent in the computer age—and it was Weese's "Rubies" that plugged in.

Darci Kistler and Kyra Nichols took turns with difficult "Diamonds." Both have performed it before, and both have recently had first babies, which is to say there is a built-in subtraction of strength. In Kistler, too much subtraction. She satisfied herself with effects (a halo here, a silvery spin there) but caught no current of sustained concentration. She now looks little, and brittle, in the face of Tchaikovsky's grandeur, unable to find herself in the fine skeins of the soliloquy or to take might from the music's ascent. Nichols, however, not as technically tight as she has been in the past, connects on ever higher levels, bringing to "Diamonds" a moving and magisterial sense of float. She's the last Balanchine ballerina on the roster, and the hush of her upper body attests to it. She's royal, Tolstoyan, unspooling arabesques and pirouettes in the white-marble corridor of Tchaikovsky's Scherzo, snow moving out of her way in drifts. She has made "Diamonds" her own lonely winter palace.

A final note. During the guild seminar, Edward Villella, who is now the artistic director of the Miami City Ballet, the only company other than NYCB ever to stage a complete *Jewels*, told how he had invited all three ballerinas—Violette Verdy, Patricia McBride, and Suzanne Farrell—to coach his ballerinas in their roles. He praised the commitment and skill of all three equally. And then he paused, angled his body toward the audience, and moved into a more searching key, as if to grapple with something difficult. It was his opinion that Suzanne had become too serious in her devotion to Balanchine, serving his memory and coaching his ballets as if she were wearing a mantle, and maybe it was too much. That Villella was compelled to voice this particular feeling, saying what has been unsaid, in the context of this particular ballet—is it not another murmur from the house of *Jewels*, a sigh from the seventh door? Farrell didn't marry Balanchine in his lifetime, but she has become the wife of his night.

March 1998

Jerome Robbins Remembered

When Jerome Robbins died on July 29, 1998, at the age of seventy-nine, the world lost not one choreographer, but two. One of these choreographers was a genius.

This was the Jerome Robbins who choreographed thirteen Broadway shows—legend among them *On the Town*, *The King and I*, *Peter Pan*, *Gypsy*, and *Fiddler on the Roof*. This was the Robbins who conceived, directed, and choreographed *West Side Story*, the musical and film phenomenon that had every baby-boomer boy in America attempting that chesty Jets leap, that T (for testosterone) in the air. And this was the Robbins of *Fancy Free*, a ballet whose character—down-to-earth, free of classical pretensions—is captured forever in its title.

In fact, *Fancy Free* was Robbins's birth cry, his *c'est moi*. Though he'd studied widely—modern dance, ethnic, and ballet in the 1930s—and had worked with the Yiddish Art Theater, it was in this comic ballet about three sailors on leave that he burst upon the scene complete, with a choreographic voice so clear and confident, so cut-to-the-chase concise that you'd never guess it was a first anything. Writing of *Fancy Free*'s 1944 premiere at American Ballet Theatre, the critic Edwin Denby said of the smash hit, "Its sentiment of how people live in this country is completely intelligent and completely realistic." More important, "The whole number is as sound as a superb vaudeville turn; in ballet terminology it is perfect American character ballet."

Fancy Free was a masterpiece of sexy-slangy storytelling—John O'Hara meets Jack Cole—and such a concentration of gesture and energy, high hopes and humor, that one year later it was actually opened out into a musical. Robbins and *Fancy Free*'s composer, a young unknown named Leonard Bernstein, along with the librettists Comden and Green, turned it into *On the Town*. Imagine, a Broadway musical born from a twenty-minute ballet.

The inverse was possible too. In 1951, for *The King and I*, Robbins choreographed "The Small House of Uncle Thomas," a dance-pantomime that pinpoints the musical's theme of slavery versus freedom. It is fixed in the musical like an exquisite bird in a golden cage, yet in memory it floats free, its own world with its own beating heart. In his heroine's escape—"run Eliza run, run from Simon"—Robbins burns that beating heart into the ear and eye. And he does this with a stress of brilliant simplicity. Eliza moves by hopping on one bare foot, the other flexed in Hinduese behind her. It is a childlike hopscotch, a crippled skip of flight, tightrope-taut within a Siamese silhouette of bent limbs and splayed fingers. Here is Robbins's poetic gift in full display, a synthesis that is kinetic and true. For sheer formal terror on the dance stage, the zigzagging bloodhounds of Simon Legree have it all over the evil fairy Carabosse of *The Sleeping Beauty*. Well, Robbins understood tyrants. He himself was a mythic monster in the studio, driving dancers into the crosshairs of his perfectionism.

Robbins went back and forth between Broadway and ballet (he choreographed a little for ABT, a lot for NYCB, where he became a ballet master in 1969), and his best work reads on any stage. In 1995, when New York City Ballet decided to present Robbins's dances from *West Side Story*—a suite he'd arranged for *Jerome Robbins' Broadway* (1988), a show of Robbins's greatest Broadway hits—there was disdain among the Kremlinologists. George Balanchine, they grumbled, had never seen fit to put these dances on his stage (he objected, I think, to boys in blue jeans). And yet *West Side Story* was the rocket blast of the 1995 season (and each season since), and not just because Robbins had rehearsed it within an inch of its life, or because the dancers brought a hot-blooded, rumbling joy to their roles as Jets, Sharks, and chicks. Robbins worked a stunning opposition into the choreography: explosive displays of sexual, territorial energy were trapped within the dynamics of popular dance (mambas, cha-chas, jazz contractions, beatnik shrugs), and so luminously constructed that you saw everything—wide shot, zoom-in, switchblade.

It was thrilling to see ballet boys in blue jeans lifting into those huge T's in their fresh T-shirts. The dances weren't arty; they weren't dated. They were vivid with social jitters to which rap kids can relate. "I would guess that in a few decades," wrote the film critic Pauline Kael in a famously scathing review of 1963, "the dances in *West Side Story* will look as much like hilariously limited, dated period pieces as Busby Berkeley's 'Remember the Forgotten Man' number in *Gold Diggers of 1933*." She guessed wrong. This is perfect American character ballet, and its audience is alive.

The other Jerome Robbins was the choreographer who turned his back on Broadway in the late 1960s. This artist was tired of the endless fight and compromise that came with any enterprise involving big-bucks egos. What Robbins wanted was to choreograph in a situation where he had sole control of the work. A ballet company offered this. He was also, I believe, searching, reaching, for a choreographic voice that had thus far eluded him, a voice that would not be qualified as "character ballet," but was classical.

What Robbins did not possess as a choreographer was apparent in his second ballet, *Interplay* (1945). It had the sort of plotless plot Robbins would return to again and again—youngish dancers joshing around, playing with classical steps in a communal bubble of vague emotional temperature. Just as Denby declared what was so bold and right about *Fancy Free*, he fingered what Robbins was missing in *Interplay*: "In point of expression he has difficulty in the complete transformation of specific pantomime images into the large and sweeping rhythm and images of direct dancing."

This is a rather abstract distinction, but what Denby means is that Robbins was grafting images onto his ballet, not drawing them out. It was synthetic versus organic. Classical dancing is its own growing language of shape, shadow, visual echoes receding, intonations blossoming. It is a language that does not require synthesis with other dance forms, though it can accommodate other forms. To see in this way is a peculiar imaginative gift—the proverbial *baiser de la fée*—and you have it or you don't. Robbins possessed the steps, adopted the classical etiquette, had formal facility to spare, and was superb within the framework of beginning, middle, and end (*The Cage*; *Afternoon of a Faun*; *The Concert*; *Ives, Songs*). But the secret meanings, the poetic infinite—this was beyond him. He had not been kissed.

But how he strived to reach that plane. There were the acclaimed, ambitious, "pure" works like *Dances at a Gathering* (1969) and *Goldberg Variations* (1971)—graceful, large-scale "interplays" to Chopin and Bach, ballets in which long length seems to speak for their seriousness. They are sleek yet slow going, beautifully fluent but not quite rich or deep. Take *Watermill*, which Robbins choreographed for Edward Villella in 1972. A presage of Robert Wilson, it is another experiment in duration, only this one a Zen time bend in which Villella hardly moves. Again, no breakthrough.

Robbins's frustrations were never more apparent than in his final collaboration with Leonard Bernstein. Balanchine's great collaborator had been Igor Stravinsky, and, in a smaller, narrower vein, Bernstein was Robbins's. The two were well aware of Balanchine and Stravinsky above them—never more so than in their work on *West Side Story*. While all the talk focused on its being a contemporary version of Shakespeare's *Romeo and Juliet*, the musical's aesthetic precedent could be found in Stravinsky. Bernstein detonated his score with the screams and implosions of *Le Sacre du printemps*, and Robbins worked the social spasms of Nijinsky's peasants into his gang dances. *West Side Story* is less a tale of love than a tale of tribes (at first, Maria was not Puerto Rican, she was Jewish).

In 1974, at NYCB, Robbins and Bernstein premiered *Dybbuk*, a ballet based on a classic of the Jewish theater, a magico-religious ghost story. In his book *Thirty Years/The New York City Ballet*, Lincoln Kirstein devotes four pages of psychoanalysis to Robbins's work on *Dybbuk*, focusing on his obsession with abstraction. "The first performance passed well enough," writes Kirstein:

> *Soon after, instead of building onto present elements, Robbins commenced cutting. It was as if he were unable to make the work "abstract" enough, as if some dybbuk were pursuing him. I admit I never saw need for abstraction. . . . While the music was drawn powerfully from*

ethnic material, and dance steps could hardly resist following Bernstein's domineering pulse, there was a constant if almost haphazard effort to strip the action of any shred of literal legibility.

It was compulsive self-sacrifice, Robbins rending his own magical storytelling, his gift, as if in some bargain with the patriarchs, an initiation rite into a mystic circle. *Dybbuk* was finally shelved because Bernstein got fed up with Robbins's changes. And Robbins, probably the wealthiest choreographer who ever lived, a success in so many wonderful ways but not the way he wanted, went on. He made a total of sixty-six ballets.

Robbins was drawn to Bach in his last years. It was not an obvious match, but Robbins seemed at home in this bubble, happy to answer that stern voice of trills and ringlets. Robbins's last ballet, *Brandenburg*, was premiered in 1997 and was again overlong, with the old coyness of *Interplay* reading faux from a choreographer of seventy-eight. Three years earlier, in 1994, Robbins made a showpiece for students at the School of American Ballet. This work, *2 & 3 Part Inventions*, took facility as its subject. Robbins paid express attention to the pointe, working the young foot the way Bach's Inventions work the young hand, finding a correspondence, a corridor, between these essential levers of creation—ten fingers, ten toes. He treated the students not as kooky kids but as young artists in search of maturity, testing technique for its poetry. Robbins's desire to the end, that searching and reaching, was a very deep bow to the art of ballet.

September 1998

Tchaikovsky at the Millennium

The overture to *Swan Lake* begins with a high F-sharp held out over a void. The tone is plaintive, isolated—a long sigh. It is on this same high, held note that Pyotr Ilyich Tchaikovsky begins his famous "swan theme," though by the time we first hear it, at the end of Act One, that tone no longer seems a sigh, but a state. This is the theme everyone hums when they hear the words *Swan Lake*, the mysterious theme, curling in a turmoil of metamorphosis, that keeps trying to vault above that opening F-sharp, which it hits three more times in four measures as if the note were a spell that must be broken. In a mere four measures, Tchaikovsky has sounded out the ballet: Odette is spellbound, a swan-woman trapped in perpetual transformation, ravishingly so. In a mere four measures, we have heard Tchaikovsky's genius for turning sound into silhouette, incantation into shape, seduction into soul. No wonder this theme was used as the overture for *Dracula* in 1931. *Swan Lake* is less a fairy tale than it is that shocking blossom of romanticism—a horror story. It is a tale of doubles and doom in the manner of Hoffmann or Coleridge or Poe.

The provenance of Tchaikovsky's first ballet, premiered in 1877, is lost in the mists of time. The names that appear on *Swan Lake*'s libretto are Begichev and Geltser, but scholars question their authorship because Tchaikovsky's fingerprints are everywhere. In his superb book *Tchaikovsky's Ballets*, Roland John Wiley points to nearby sources such as a folktale by Musäus called *The Swans' Pond*, and, more compellingly, Wagner's opera *Lohengrin*, in which a white swan figures symbolically. Tchaikovsky admired *Lohengrin*, calling it "the crown of Wagner's creations."

It isn't just Wagner's opera, however, that Wiley detects in Tchaikovsky's ballet, but Tchaikovsky's own earlier operas—*Undine* (1869) and *Mandragora* (1870)—as well as his incidental music for *The Snow Maiden* (1873). All share the same scenario, the tragic love between a non-mortal woman and a mortal man. "Tchaikovsky destroyed *Undine* and abandoned *Mandragora*," writes Wiley. "It is possible that he perceived in *Swan Lake* a vehicle more satisfactory than the others to present this kind of love story, which he seemed to find so attractive." In a kind of transmutation, the love duet from *Undine* would become the Act Two lakeside pas de deux in *Swan Lake*.

And then there is the living-room ballet called *The Lake of the Swans*, which Tchaikovsky created for family entertainments at least five years before he began work on *Swan Lake*. "The staging of the ballet was done entirely by Pyotr Ilyich," remembered Tchaikovsky's nephew Yury Lvovich Davydov. "It was he who invented the steps and pirouettes, and he danced them himself, showing the performers what he required of them . . . as he sang the tune." Furthermore, according to Davydov, "the principal theme—'The Song of the Swans'—was then the same as now." This is not so much a fingerprint as a potent piece of DNA.

What we know for sure is that a score like *Swan Lake*'s was utterly new to ballet. Its orchestral depth and richness, tonalities like layers of consciousness, and dramatic wholeness inspired musicologists to deem it the first "symphonic" ballet. But it also contains the sinuous inner contours of opera—narrow paths, fates unfolding, voices. "Take any pas de deux," George Balanchine has said of *Swan Lake*, "their melodies are absolutely vocal." In *Swan Lake*, Tchaikovsky plumbed the singing line for mass and space, tempered it for embodiment. *Swan Lake* is the first ballet score in which we feel rapt corporeal presence, psychosexual weight. It's a ballet Freud could put on the couch and analyze.

Indeed, *Swan Lake* is a cliff-drop into sensuality, and Odette looks like no other creature in ballet. Giselle may become undead but she is never less than human. The Sylph is made of air and wing, but she was formed in man's image. Tchaikovsky's Swan Queen, however . . . what is she? Swan by day, human by night, her clock akin to the vampire's? Or is she a hybrid of woman and bird, something like the

Landscape with Moving Figures

Fly? Is she the Ideal as Escape? Sublimation as the Sublime? No one knows and no one need know. She is Tchaikovsky—an F-sharp tense within a melody that arches like a swan's neck, aches like a question mark. She is the sound of desire.

In Tchaikovsky's own life, desire was a subject increasingly fraught. In his definitive biography, *Tchaikovsky: The Quest for the Inner Man*, Alexander Poznansky explains that while Tchaikovsky was a confirmed and generally guilt-free homosexual, he nevertheless knew that his sexual preference made him and his loved ones vulnerable to dangerous gossip. In 1876, the year he composed *Swan Lake*, fears of blackmail, however exaggerated, were swirling in his head. He began toying with the idea of marriage, thinking a nod to convention would secure a zone of protection around his name and work. In early May 1877, less than three months after the premiere of *Swan Lake* and a few weeks before he started work on the opera *Eugene Onegin*, Tchaikovsky began courting the music student Antonina Milyukova. By the end of May he had proposed a *mariage blanc*. She married without understanding, and then expected—to his horror, despair, disgust—the real thing. It was over (unconsummated) in two months, at which point Tchaikovsky began referring to Milyukova as "the reptile."

Explaining it later, Tchaikovsky (and his biographer-peers) liked to imply that he was caught up in the heady parallels between Onegin and himself, Tatiana and Antonina. Poznansky views this as wishful thinking. And there is a better parallel. *Swan Lake* is about a disastrous marriage, a prince who out of duty must wed, finds an otherworldly soulmate in the strange white swan Odette (*mariage blanc!*), and then mistakenly makes a vow of love to the black swan Odile, the evil, rather reptilian, double of Odette. It's not a perfect parallel. To begin with, the prince in *Swan Lake* is deceived by Von Rothbart and Odile, whereas Tchaikovsky essentially deceived himself. But like his marriage, *Swan Lake* is a flower of his fears, the creature from his black lagoon. Tchaikovsky's twilight anxieties—a longing for resolve, a pervasive mistrust—are at home in these reeds and waters.

Swan Lake has ghoulish trappings—old stone castles, a shape-shifting villain (Von Rothbart, who takes the form of a bat or owl)—but the ballet is usually produced prettily, with storybook simplicity.

Last season, Matthew Bourne's *Swan Lake*, an import from England, plundered the sexual subtext and became a pop phenomenon with an extended run on Broadway. Recasting *Swan Lake* with a gender twist, Bourne turned up the gothic high dudgeon, giving us a story of sexual hysteria set in Buckingham Palace. The prince—love-starved, hungry for something—ends in madness, a sort of self-immolation by swan.

Bourne's *Swan Lake* is not a ballet. It is a giddy piece of theater masquerading as dance. In the manner of Mark Morris's *The Hard Nut*, which set *The Nutcracker* in an acidic sixties suburb, Bourne's production is an update: party dances are the Twist and the Frug, though the Queen Mum still wears pinch-waist silhouettes from the fifties. The staging is impressive, continuously clever, with the overscaled prop from one scene gliding and revolving to unlock the next scene, like objects floating through a dream retold. And in the lakeside "white acts," Bourne makes the story his own. Act Two is a London park of white-plaster surrealism, very Cecil Beaton in *Vogue*—a gay wink. Act Four is a white straitjacket in a white room—shock-therapy apotheosis.

The big gimmick in this production is that the swans are danced by bare-chested men in woolly (why not feathers?) white bloomers and punk makeup. Odette might be thought of as a Mapplethorpe orchid, a multi-cult Other, while Odile is rough trade in black leather, a bisexual threat. For a while, the spectacle of powdered pecs and powerful arms is fascinating—the male weight rocks the score like an overloaded boat. And always, when a stage is full of raw young men moving as one, there is that communal, feral thrill in the audience, a cheap thrill, but potent in its moment. The point where the choreography should be most inventive—the swans—is where invention falls away. Bourne has deftly cut the score elsewhere, but it sounds as if he's used every last drop of the white acts. This leaves a lot of time to see that his swan steps are modern-dance pastiche, mostly waist up and heavily repetitive. The erotic charge quickly goes flat—okay, flap-flap, boy swans. The strangeness is not where it should be, in the steps.

I admit to a gut reaction against Bourne's vision of the swan as male. Yes, there is a rush in the score dynamic enough to support masculine muscle. But Bourne's *Swan Lake* does not, cannot, sing. Tchaikovsky understood ballerinas, and was known to do fair imitations of them. His feathery orchestrations speak to slim female ankles and delicate wrists. His slides up the scale beg for the trill of finger turns and pirouettes on pointe. And his adagios, like a soprano's arias (that F-sharp is soprano range), are at one with the lengthening of line made possible by women's pointe work and deep plié (men do not lift any higher than demi-pointe, nor do they articulate plié with as much roundness and refinement). Lev Ivanov, choreographer of the 1895 Mariinsky white acts that have remained the template for stagings ever since, responded to Tchaikovsky with metaphors—shapes that nest in space, steps *en tournant* in which the two-sided spell (day/night) seems to reverberate ad infinitum. Bourne's muscle-beach birds haven't the existential poetry of women, the corps as state of grace or moaning mass grave.

Still, conventional *Swan Lake*s are harder and harder to sit through. Clichés of staging have grown thick and predictable (all those pleasant peasants), the national dances look tediously rote, and no one seems to know what to do with that storm-swept Act Four where Tchaikovsky, lashing toward death and transcendence under a rising astral canopy, overwhelms most attempts at staging (Bourne's best stroke was his imploding finale—he makes it an electrical brainstorm, horror-story hyperbole). Regarding Odette, today's ballerinas think they know her. They think she is a white tutu, a flutter of arms, a tragic face. You no longer feel them sinking into her arched-back attitudes as into abyss, the way Natalia Makarova used to do. You no longer feel them plunged into that sacrificial plastique, the imprisoned arabesques and *soutenus*. Eloquently helpless, sadistically enchanted, sullied yet pure— Odette is like Garbo's throat, a place or grace that is beyond the pale of today's Gen X female imagination. She is a daughter of adagio, that magisterial elaboration of line, which in its continuous pull between arrest and movement builds a monument to emotion. In scoring Odette's themes for the reedy oboe, Tchaikovsky was clear about the struggle on his mind: she is sucked down by the marshes even as she reaches for the moon.

In his *Swan Lake* of 1951, George Balanchine was right to dispense with the court, the plot, the national dances. "I remember when *Swan Lake* was performed at the Mariinsky Theatre," he says in *Balanchine's Tchaikovsky*, a book of interviews with Solomon Volkov, "*no one ever understood anything!*" [His italics.] Balanchine elided Acts Two and Four into a fantasia of *Swan Lake*, dropping the ballerina into a blue current that swept her up and away.

What would he have thought of last spring's *Swan Lake* at New York City Ballet? Probably what everybody thought: Why? As part of the company's fiftieth-anniversary season, this new production by Peter Martins read like a non sequitur; it was everything Balanchine had attempted to forgo with his own concentrated version. Coming on the heels of Bourne's *Swan Lake*, with its theatrical brio, its full-frontal eros, Martins's work looked dispassionate, flat, no sex drive at all. It's as if he himself were playing the prince, forced by duty into a loveless marriage with *Swan Lake*.

There isn't much good to say about the production. Per Kirkeby's sets were minimal suggestions of place, and the few props—a crossbow on a pillow, a throne—had the bright, static look of icons on a computer screen. While the lakeside acts were blue-gray Silly String abstractions, Act Three, a looming, wood-paneled room, could have been office space for a CEO. Around Ivanov's heated duets and solos, Martins supplied the kind of cold, fast, dancers-in-endless-lines-of-four choreography he does to the music of Michael Torke and Charles Wuorinen.

Into this empty exercise came the company's unprepared Odette-Odiles. Some tried squeezing into the swan's introverted, curve-on-curve plastique (Monique Meunier kept popping out of it, as if her stays wouldn't hold). Others sort of skimmed along the top, connecting the solos. What else could they do? You can't just put on that tutu and be Odette in a full-length production. It takes layers of commitment—emotional, technical, communal—to the style and the story. The style *is* the story. But it's just an outline to these women, not in their tradition. You can see they don't know how to make it theirs, and consequently they have no love for it. In fact, Martins actually choreographed this *Swan Lake* for the Royal Danish Ballet, where it was premiered a year ago. Why it was deemed appropriate for the New York City Ballet is a mystery not of the lakeside but of the boardroom.

The Sleeping Beauty, Tchaikovsky's second ballet, is also about a marriage, also fixed on the continuation of the royal line, but what a different marriage it is. Premiered in 1890, thirteen years after *Swan Lake*, *Beauty* is like day to *Swan Lake's* night. You hear the difference at once in the overtures. Where *Swan Lake* is a lone voice floating in darkness, *Sleeping Beauty* begins in discourse: the ripping cry and kettledrum rumble of the furious fairy Carabosse is answered and subdued by the calm breeze and harp glissandos of the Lilac Fairy. Where *Swan Lake's* overture builds with the throb of obsession, in *Beauty* we experience the social fabric—torn, then mended—of the true fairy tale. It's difficult not to feel an almost ontological force at work in these two scores. *Swan Lake* sounds like a ballet conceived in mist and composed in isolation. *Beauty* is the blossom of a close, committed, and well-documented collaboration between Tchaikovsky and the masters of the Mariinsky Ballet—the director Ivan Vsevolozhsky and the choreographer Marius Petipa. In short, *Sleeping Beauty* is a marriage of like minds.

The idea was Vsevolozhsky's. He was keen on a collaboration between Tchaikovsky, Petipa, and himself, but his first proposal, *Undine*, didn't interest Tchaikovsky (who may have felt he'd been there, done that). The scenario Vsevolozhsky prepared from Charles Perrault's *La Belle au bois dormant*, however, charmed the Francophile in all three men (though French, Petipa thought himself a Russian artist). "I want to do the mise en scène in Louis XIV style," Vsevolozhsky wrote. "Here one could let one's musical fantasy run wild and compose melodies in the spirit of Lully, Bach, Rameau, etc." It would be a sumptuous production, a *ballet-féerie* set in Versailles. But more than that, *Beauty* would be a supreme integration of aesthetic affinities—musical, theatrical, epochal—with seventeenth- and eighteenth-century ideals recapitulated in nineteenth-century forms, and lyric flight (the troubadour's rose) absorbed into classical amplitude (the Baroque sunburst). Beginning in the era of Louis XIV, the Sun King, and ending in the clouds of Apollo, the Sun God, the ballet is framed in light and offers an implicit, flattering portrait of Russia's Czar Alexander III, who was footing the bill. Implicit as well was a bold territorial statement: *Beauty* suggests it was the Russian Ballet—not French—that was now continuing the line of classical dance.

Petipa wrote up a detailed choreo-musical libretto (in the Vision Scene coda, for example, he wants "music with mutes—a 2/4 as in *A Midsummer Night's Dream*"), and Tchaikovsky responded with a masterpiece that is its own dreaming kingdom, a score not easily altered or rearranged. Tchaikovsky's light touch shows the influence not of Lully but of Delibes's *Coppélia* and *Sylvia*, ballets Tchaikovsky had come to know only after he wrote *Swan Lake*. And he'd made another adjustment. Gone the Sturm und Drang of Wagner; the operatic model for *Beauty* is the self-contained, human-scaled, witty, and forgiving opera of Tchaikovsky's god, Mozart. In *Beauty*, sensuality is not dangerously concentrated in one being (contrary to Odette in *Swan Lake*), it is in the order of the material world, touching all things. Tchaikovsky's score—the rapture of its orchestral colors, the splendor of its suspension-bridge structure, its melodies like little vignettes and long vistas—is a realm where characters fall and grow, where the senses graduate into sensibility. *The Sleeping Beauty* is an Enlightenment ballet.

For Wiley, the score makes brilliant choices tantamount to a philosophical statement. In *Swan Lake*, keys are locked in opposition, searching in vain for resolution. But in *Beauty*, the principal keys "have no commanding interrelationship beyond their compatibility with the key of resolution [G]," to which all these keys lead. Furthermore, "In *Sleeping Beauty*, Tchaikovsky chooses E minor and E major to portray the malevolent and benevolent aspects of Aurora's destiny, personified by Carabosse and the Lilac Fairy . . . they are quite different, yet in some respects the same." Good and evil, life and death, E-ternally bound—this, too, is in the order of things. Such balances in the story and the score, embodied in Aurora's famous balances in the Rose Adagio, make *Beauty* the lyric expression of a cherished hope: that good does subdue evil, that humankind will always right itself. This is why *Beauty* is beloved, why that first production bound so many young artists—Anna Pavlova, Léon Bakst, and later George Balanchine—to ballet. In *The Sleeping Beauty*, civilization is an art, and art, a civilization. This is why the Royal Ballet's *Beauty* of 1946, with Margot Fonteyn as Aurora, had such a profound impact. After so much death, it looked like dawn.

Landscape with Moving Figures

But what did the first *Sleeping Beauty* look like? You can imagine the excitement among balletomanes when it was learned that the Kirov Ballet, now under the direction of Makhar Vaziev, was reconstructing the 1890 *Beauty*. Memories of a *Beauty* the company brought to New York in 1989 had, for me, dwindled to a felt hat with a curling feather, a vine-covered scrim, a slow evening of powder pastels. That was a *Beauty* of patchy provenance, a long way and a few revolutions from Vsevolozhsky and Petipa, though compared to shiny American *Beauty*s the old-world dustiness had charm. This new—or rather, new-old—*Beauty* was the result of a chance comment the American scholar Tim Scholl made to Vaziev, "Have you seen the Sergeyev notes?" He was referring to the extensive notations that Nikolai Sergeyev had made of Petipa's *Sleeping Beauty* at the beginning of the century, notations that were asleep in the Harvard Theatre Collection. (A second Sergeyev—Konstatin—ran the Kirov from the 1950s through the 1970s, and made his own changes to *Beauty* in those years.)

For a blow-by-blow story of the restoration, go to *Ballet Review*, Spring 1999, where the mapping and weighing of Nikolai Sergeyev's notes, the matching of his steps and floor plans against old memories and even older *Beauty*s, is fascinating aesthetic detective work. Meanwhile, the reports from visitors to Russia were raves. There were also backstage politics. Russian dancers traditionally don't like to try new things, even new-old things. The senior dancers didn't like this *Beauty* because it wasn't their *Beauty*, and the younger dancers didn't like the wigs. The long blond Louis Quinze curls Prince Désiré wears in Act Two almost bit the dust when one dancer refused to wear them (he relented, when the other dancer cast as Désiré said *he'd* wear the wig). At the end of June, the Kirov Ballet of the Mariinsky Theatre unveiled its restored *Sleeping Beauty* at the Met.

The first chills came with the first strokes of the overture. Under the baton of Gianandrea Noseda, the Kirov Ballet Orchestra tore into Tchaikovsky—swift, fierce, ascendant—taking full possession of the music not by right of long lineage, but by the feline vigor and acute sensitivity with which it inhabited Tchaikovsky's world of sounds. This wasn't going to be one of those stately *Beauty*s. In seconds, the audience was sitting up straighter, all the better to see the sights.

The lovely sepia-tinted archival photos in the souvenir program—Aurora in amber—simply didn't prepare one for the clash of colors when the curtain went up: yellows, violets, turquoise, emerald green (later, chlorine green in the Vision Scene), not to mention gold and silver, pearls and embroideries, sashes and plumes. The artist Alexander Benois, there at the beginning, thought the combination of costume colors garish, and it is, vibrantly, vibratingly. We are now so conditioned to seeing color-coordinated productions of the classics, so used to equating authenticity or relevance with a homogenized facade, we feel adrift when we don't get that facade (and then vaguely disappointed when we do). The life force of these colors was a revelation, and not lost on the crowd.

The sets stick with Vsevolozhsky's plan of Versailles-like courts, bedchambers, gardens, and forests. But within architectural backdrops full of ornate play, trompe l'oeil vaults and niches, Vsevolozhsky had a field day with the costumes. The corsetted, bustled, *tapissier* (upholsterer) style of the couturier Charles Worth, who had dressed Empress Eugénie, is used for the Lilac Fairy's Act Two costume and Princess Aurora's wedding gown, linking them in divine right, and also keeping them fashionably up-to-date (the other court ladies are back with Louis in abbreviated panniers). And what about those red-and-white striped tights like gondola poles—stripes everywhere!—and the explosion of plackets and pom-poms? Tim Scholl has noted that St. Petersburg connoisseurs were then under the spell of the commedia dell'arte. Vsevolozhsky mixed fantasy and fact, centuries and styles, with the cheek of Diana Vreeland.

Four hours long, this *Beauty* flies by. It is divided into four short acts with three intermissions, as American Ballet Theatre's currently is. Yet it never feels heavy, as ABT's does. One of the glories of this production is its easy sense of time. Petipa opens the prologue with pageantry and pantomime, taking special care to make relationships clear. He's telling the story, and the dances that follow simply open that story to the atmosphere. When the fairies promenade in with their entourages, the party begins. When the fairies dance, a magic, almost psychedelic, garden is born onstage. This swing between

Landscape with Moving Figures

forms of expression makes for a metaphysical balance, a luxurious pace, a magical mystery tour that's never slow.

This marvelous pace allows us time to use our eyes, to see more. For instance, I love the way the solo of the Wheat Flour Fairy is followed, of course, by the Breadcrumbs Fairy, who has mice appliquéd on her tutu, wanting their share of crumbs. Who's next but a bird, the Canary Fairy. In Vsevolozhsky and Petipa's kingdom even the crumbs connect. And when the big bad fairy Carabosse storms the party, moving with humpbacked menace, it's a black cat that adorns her cape. The cat and mouse in the costumes is just another of the eternal circles in this *Beauty*.

On a deeper level, the material richness of the production connects with one of its primary choreographic metaphors—not the image of the rose, central to the ballet and redolent of Aurora, but its sister image, the spindle. Both spiral around a stem or axis, both have sharp points, both evoke a ballerina up on pointe. But where the rose suggests one, the spindle suggests the interweaving, the interdependence, of many. And like a sewing needle appearing and disappearing in cloth, the idea of the point—not only its danger but its power—keeps flashing in this *Beauty*, reiterated in its props: knitting needles, the Lilac Fairy's silver sword, Prince Désiré's arrow. Everyone, this production seems to say, has a point.

Petipa put ample space around his pointes. In one of the production's striking reversions, the Lilac Fairy's big solo in the prologue no longer consists of those grand, horizon-like leg sweeps that no one can quite do these days. Instead, it's a series of beautifully modeled *passés* which, once you get used to it, is more syntactically compatible with Aurora's solos, their Singer sewing machine verticality and precision, their *piqué* (pricked) footwork. More interesting still is Petipa's continual return to attitude *en avant*, the leg hooked in front of the body. He uses it again and again, usually angled *croisé*, so much that it becomes as important as attitude *derrière*—the pose of Mercury that is Aurora's signature pose and the iconic focus of productions ever since. Attitude *en avant* acts as a little gate to the stage, a thornlike protection of Tchaikovsky's kingdom (surely these attitudes were an influence on Frederick Ashton). It also presents the pointe on a pillow of air.

If the body's rise and fall is fixed in the pointed toe, pantomime and dance meet in the pointed finger. It is employed everywhere in Petipa's *Beauty*: by the fairies for sculptural finish; by Carabosse to spell fate; by Aurora to show her wound; and by Lilac, who taps her forehead to say, "Think." This *Beauty* passes from fingertip to fingertip to fingertip, a golden thread of artistic impulse and inspiration.

Of the many adorable touches in this *Beauty*, one stands out. At the end of the Prologue, having cast the spell of death on Aurora (only to have it softened by Lilac), Carabosse is leaving. As her carriage pulls away, all the fairies and courtiers crowd after her, their backs to the audience, all wagging a finger high in the air. Writing in the *New York Times*, Anna Kisselgoff sniffed, "It is hard to believe that Petipa would have the King and the entire court waving a finger at Carabosse." Is it? I find it hard to believe that this thrilling moment, so poetically true to the texture of the whole, so palpably Petipa, was ever allowed to go missing. "It will not be," they seem to say, and there is no moment in all of ballet so full of its own unity. By the way, in his detailed research on the first production, Wiley comes to the Prologue's end and writes, "All present threaten Carabosse."

How does the Kirov look in this *Beauty*? Like the dancers understand it, despite their qualms. They perform mime with such largesse it makes you happy. You feel the shape of the story fitting large inside the ballet—a sort of silent-movie scale—and it's utterly involving, especially today, when stories are no longer shown or told, just implied, assumed. Perhaps another circle is coming around. With the sensations of robo-dancer speed and flexibility becoming ever more thin and undifferentiated, it is human rhythm that looks new and fresh.

As for Aurora, ever since the touchstone performances of Margot Fonteyn, and later the Kirov's Irina Kolpakova and Alla Sizova, critics have looked to this role as privileged and definitive, and also as an indicator of company health—Aurora as annual report. Given the symbolisms in the ballet, it's tempting to view the role this way, but it can mar one's enjoyment of *Beauty*. A born Aurora—a new future—doesn't come along every day. It's well to remember that St. Petersburg balletomanes thought the first Aurora, Italian ballerina

Carlotta Brianza, a "little brown imp." This production made me see *Beauty* as the ensemble work it is, the little kingdom that is every classical ballet company.

The Kirov is currently in a youthful phase, with a batch of new ballerinas fresh out of the gate. Svetlana Zakharova had opening night. Long, slim, exceedingly flexible, with a smiling porcelain-doll face, she's the company ingenue. Zakharova's tendency toward trick extensions, legs flipped up mindlessly high, can make her gauche, but her upper body, the curvaceous modeling of her head, shoulders, and back, is lyric. Diana Vishneva's Aurora was deeper, more musically aware and daring (even impulsive; there's a touch of wildness in Vishneva). The way she arched soulfully sideways to drop her handful of roses—echoing, one critic noted, the handle of a basket—was Russian poetry, and an example of the unusually soft finish she likes to put on a phrase. (Later in the week, her Act Two in *Giselle* was softness on softness, again with daring musical accents like jags of unbound energy.) Altynai Asylmuratova had the matinee, not quite the place for the woman who was the company princess only ten years ago. But ten years can be a lifetime in ballet. She is weaker in the lower body (which was never technically strong), but above, majestic, poised. She is harder, with a snap of sell on her finishes, but also absolutely clear, showing the social flow of Aurora's attentions. Her arabesque is still mighty, and now weighty. It centers her in the story, and gives her grandeur.

When asked why the company took on this restoration of *The Sleeping Beauty*, Sergei Vikharev, the dancer who restaged it, told *Ballet Review*, "It's not a question of whether the current [Konstantin Sergeyev] version suits us or not, but of what is now called *The Sleeping Beauty* at the Mariinsky. Does it have anything to do with Tchaikovsky or Petipa? Should the Theatre even use their names in its programs?" Self-questioning at the Kirov? This is an amazing development. So too the company's dancing of Balanchine, as it showed in its all-Balanchine evenings at the Met. Not only was he performed without petulance, but faster, looser, lighter, and, in the dancing of Uliana Lopatkina in *Symphony in C*, phrased (good god), *embraced* in phrasing. It was the second movement renewed—and in the slow *penchée*, no tacky nose touched to knee, but measure, breath, a rose opening. A complete surprise from this usually steely ballerina, the performance made one, for the first time, think, They have all of Balanchine before them.

And they have Tchaikovsky, which is everything.

September 1999

Two Princes and a Mock Tudor

Neither American Ballet Theatre nor the New York City Ballet did anything millennial for their spring 2000 seasons at Lincoln Center, and that's a blessing, because neither American Ballet Theatre nor the New York City Ballet is in a position to do anything definitive right now. American Ballet Theatre is deep into blockbuster mentality—a kind of denial, really—whereby we get week after week of full-length story ballets (five *Taming of the Shrew*s, for example, followed by eight *La Bayadère*s), long stretches separated by two to three days of under-rehearsed repertory programs. Across the plaza, NYCB looks just joyless, as if the strain of survival in a boom-rich, arts-fickle New York, plus the immense legacy of George Balanchine, is too oppressive a load to cart into the next century. ABT is bottom heavy and ramshackle; NYCB is thin and rattled. At both, top-tier female dancers are aging or injured, with no great push coming up from underneath, and day-to-day performance has all the consistency of a marble in a pinball machine.

For the past few seasons, the light—the *tilt!*—at Lincoln Center has come from two young men at ABT: Ethan Stiefel, an elegant Apollonian blond, and Angel Corella, a boyish brunette with a burning happiness onstage. Like Hamlet and Fortinbras, both are princes, but physically, chemically different. Cast in the same roles on different nights, facing the same challenges, these two have been the show within a show at ABT, a match game score for score. Who'll dominate in *Push Comes to Shove*? Who in *Billy the Kid*? It's the best kind of competition, not only because it is an even match (in the days when Mikhail Baryshnikov technically outstripped all the other men there were no even matches), but also because both dancers have innate taste. Neither guy wants to win ugly, so everybody wins.

Stiefel was produced by the School of American Ballet and rose to principal dancer at New York City Ballet, a young man with musical daring and a rapier technique going for the big moves. He has a clear line like a quill pen in a beautiful hand moving across the page—a graceful continuity even though he has a rather tight-knit physique. His i's are dotted, his t's crossed, and Lord his toes are pointed. Stiefel left NYCB meticulously finished, yet the finish never got the better of the phrase. He was a golden boy, with round baby blues much like Baryshnikov's but a lighter, sweeter touch, something between Leonardo DiCaprio and Brad Pitt.

Stiefel joined ABT in 1997, already refined. Angel Corella came into the company with more bottom on him (literally and figuratively), two years before Stiefel. A corps dancer in Spain, he was spotted in a ballet competition in Paris (spinning, no doubt) and was taken up by ABT, where he was promptly dropped into Balanchine's *Theme and Variations*, the ABT rite of passage into which all men with potential get dropped like fledglings over a choppy sea. It's fly or swim or sink—flying's best. Corella was a little chunky in those days, a little thick through the leg, but so game, so charmingly eager to please, and to please through dancing. Watching him *not* let go of a multiple pirouette, hanging on to the spin while losing his center, I thought, Another tousle-haired tornado. I preferred Vladimir Malakhov, who also joined ABT in 1995, a dancer of long-limbed articulation and nocturnal glow.

But there is no second-guessing desire, especially when it is buttressed by discipline. And it's easier to improve alignment than it is to amp up the passion (again, Baryshnikov's a case in point: he never could make his perfection look passionate; the harder he tried, the stagier he got). Corella was making the right choice, and by his third year at ABT his technique was catching up with his heart. The arrival of Stiefel didn't hurt.

The two dancers first went memorably head to head in 1998, in the company's production of *Le Corsaire*. A Mariinsky-vintage piece of ballet exotica (beautiful Greek girls are sold in the square, then

Landscape with Moving Figures

rescued by their pirate boyfriends), *Le Corsaire* is today a choreographic hodgepodge that contains priceless nuggets of Petipa—one of them the iconographic *Corsaire* pas de deux, the slave and lady dance that famously framed Rudolf Nureyev for the public eye. Performing it with tea-finger Margot Fonteyn, he flexed, he coiled, he threw himself in spasm at her feet. It was Russia wowing the West, Rudi bent on arousal, slave to the audience (and enslaving the audience in return). Stiefel, however, likes to give contained, structured performances, and he danced the role with gleaming self-effacement, a dark gleam, making of himself a burnished totem. Corella compressed even further, curling deeper, kneeling lower. But more trusting of abandon, he opened at the top, let himself tear loose in quick synaptic riptides. Stiefel brought the house down. Corella carried it away.

In spring 1999 all eyes were on the ABT revival of *Push Comes to Shove*, Twyla Tharp's 1976 hit vehicle for Baryshnikov, a role for him to show off in. It's a curious piece, a portrait of Misha that's really a portrait of ABT's dependence on Misha as an attraction, an energy source, a bright, sharp focus. Tharp showed a certain disdain for the women around him; they're dippy, kooky, wobble-bodied. He's the crack smart-ass, and also "beauty like a tightened bow." The man who steps into this role must have the reverb of that bow, and be the arrow too. He has to be taut, shooting, heightened at once, otherwise the jokes don't fly. My money was on Stiefel.

But it was Corella who had the edge. Stiefel danced *Push* like a long classical variation (albeit one with snotty asides), giving every step 100 percent, fully stretched, fully pointed, and wearing himself out fast by holding on too hard, not winging along. It was a heroic performance in which Stiefel's good faith got in the way. *Push* is to some extent a bad-faith ballet. Its energies are those of the stand-up comic: aggressive, antisocial, out of control. This guy (a far cry from Rudi in *Corsaire*) uses the audience as a reflection in which to check his hair (and then he gives the audience an "up yours"). Corella—relaxed, class clownish, but zapping the steps—rode his own virtuosity like it was something silly.

The next face-off was *Billy the Kid*, Eugene Loring's back-pocket masterpiece of 1938, a brilliant collaboration with Aaron Copland, who turned in a haunted score that cleared space for a haunting ballet. *Billy* has been out of ABT rep for quite some time, permission revoked, I heard, because ABT performances were not up to snuff. It returned in 1999, part of the fall season at City Center. "*Billy* is about the West as it is dreamed of," the critic Edwin Denby wrote in 1943, "as it is imagined by boys playing in empty lots in the suburbs of our cities." The make-believe of kids playing is on a continuum with the make-believe of ballet.

Little Billy sustains big performances because he's like Don Giovanni—the one with the energy, the one you root for. But the energy has to stay sharply inside the stylized lines, resonating within those dandy costumes (eye-popping black-and-white stripes, then little-kid stars). Corella tends to be more rapt than concentrated. He's riveted to the stage world around him, hearing, seeing, and as Billy he kicks into the role with his little black boots, his big brown eyes innocent of his own brutality. It was a jangly portrayal, as if Corella's spurs were loose (his cowboy hat really was loose, slipping down over those puppy eyes), but held together by charisma. In this ballet, though, charisma doesn't beat concentration. Stiefel sank into Billy as if it were a character role, affecting a bowlegged walk and a bitter grimace. His Billy was a conscious killer, heavy with hate—a risky path on Stiefel's part, a fine line between character and cartoon, but it was the right line, his portrayal having the impacted power of Philip Guston's one-eyed wedges. And then there was the tenderness he brought to the duet in the desert, when Billy is thinking of his sweetheart (who is an echo of his mother). Billy is meant to be alone, imagining, so Stiefel performs the entire duet looking beyond his partner, and suddenly Billy is weightless, as if he's dancing with the stars in the backdrop. It's a glimpse behind the mask, unbearably sad.

The fascinating thing about Stiefel and Corella is that their side-by-side ascent has galvanized them at a time when other ABT principals are looking undirected, lost, or "lite." Vladimir Malakhov, gifted, vivid in his first years with the company, has somehow marginalized himself, giving performances of empty elegance, his phosphorescence on the fritz. His gala night performance of *Tchaikovsky Pas de Deux*, the Balanchine showstopper, set the tone. He danced it bouncing like a baby, as if it were Bournonville, as wrong as wrong can be. Where is his coach? Does he have one? Julie Kent, once a dancer of delicacy and moonlight, has gotten grande dame-ish, exerting a Margot Fonteyn-like pretty-pretty reign over the repertory, and giving herself airs by dancing roles she has no business putting a foot in, like the season's first week *Theme and Variations*. Kent was a shambles—slow, blurred, hoisted around by her poor partner, not strong or sharp enough to cut the crystal. Mid-season she practically walked through *Jardin aux Lilas* ("Lilac Garden"), once one of her most glowing roles. And by the final week's *Manon* pas de deux with Julio Bocca, she was cheating with a lot of head and neck action, lascivious glances flashed at the audience. *Manon* is slippery and Kent is square, a dancer boxed in by her correctness and pleased to be in that box, getting boxier with every year. She needs to trade her airs for oxygen.

And Ashley Tuttle. This dancer has been slow to blossom, so slow she always strikes me as older than she is. She has the older dancer's love of adagio, and in the slow spells of *La Bayadère* or *Giselle* or *Theme and Variations* she's like a white goldfish drifting, lilting, alone in a glass globe. Her soul bubble is wonderful, and then suddenly it's not, she's too far away. It doesn't help that she's pinched through the hips, and so lacks freedom, swing, getting her legs up and around. She's too young to be so circumscribed. Is it an injury, bad training? Tuttle has a ballerina's wayward sense of invention, but her technical problems tamp down her impact, holding her to a middling scale, more soloist than star.

As for Stiefel and Corella this spring, Stiefel—wearing a feather and turquoise harem pants as Ali, the slave in *Le Corsaire*—graced the billboards in front of the Met, but was out for the entire season with mononucleosis. And Corella—I'm not surprised—was lackluster. It began on the first night, the gala, when he danced the *Corsaire* pas de deux and finished his phrases with that hard hand-snap of dispatch. That snap is running rampant through ABT, a coarse punctuation that may feel necessary in the cavernous Met space (it's not), and is also a covering tactic for dancers tired or just plain weak

Two Princes and a Mock Tudor

(it covers nothing). Feet flap, fouettés falter, pirouettes go *pfffft*, but the dancers meet the end of the phrase like snapping banners—"I did it!"—even though they didn't. It was disconcerting to see Corella selling *Corsaire*, but in every Corella performance I saw this season—James in *La Sylphide*, Solor in *La Bayadère*, even the Lover in *Jardin aux Lilas*—he put a weird whippy finish on his phrases. It's hard not to feel that Stiefel's sterling sensibility holds Corella to a higher standard of refinement, just as Corella's bliss in virtuosity is a spur to Stiefel. It has always been said that ABT dancers have to do it themselves. It is lately said, as well, that a lot of ABT coaching is now done "by compliment," meaning the principals get more coddling than criticism. We all know where that leads. It leads to Julie Kent making mash of *Theme* (or even being in *Theme*), to Paloma Herrera dancing the *Corsaire* pas de deux as if she were in a circus, center ring. It leads to dancing that doesn't look like a product of anything, or in the plaintive words of a fellow critic, "They have no kinetic depth."

The new *Swan Lake* that ABT artistic director Kevin McKenzie staged and premiered this season, a 1.5 million-dollar baby, is certainly attractive with its Roseville colors, its Rookwood trees. It's also up-to-date, with borrowings from Matthew Bourne's Broadway version of *Swan Lake*, including Bourne's stress on sexual thralldom (in McKenzie's Act Three, Von Rothbart openly seduces the visiting princesses). And I liked the shock-lit Frankenstein landscape of Act Four, a minute of originality. Otherwise, this *Swan Lake* is all set and no sensibility, with nothing palpably ABT about it. And something palpable is exactly the point. *Swan Lake*, perhaps more than any other ballet, is about kinetic logic, which is the life force of a ballet company, a systemic poetic force coursing through all its shapes and forms. Unlike the Kirov or the Royal or the Bolshoi (which even at extremely low ebb, as the company was in its visit this summer, still works as one with that turned-in, high-hearted push); unlike NYCB where the issue of kinetic logic—how a dancer moves, how the company dances—is one of the crucial aesthetic issues of our time; unlike these great companies, ABT does not have a school feeding into the corps and is therefore not coherent from the ground up. Company class, coaches, and critically attuned choreography must face these aesthetic differences, must forge, at least, an ethic, a standard.

In his long career, George Balanchine never stopped commenting on the innate laziness of the human body, how with dancers you had to "start pushing them and scream at them to make them more alive." It was high praise to be "not bad." Antony Tudor, who made masterpieces for ABT during his nearly five-decade association with the company, and whose ballets sound the deepest chords in ABT history, was notoriously blunt and manipulative with dancers, his mind games the stuff of lore. He did not choreograph or coach by compliment. What would Tudor say if he saw this season's performances of his ballet *Jardin aux Lilas*? ABT used to be definitive in Tudor.

Jardin aux Lilas was choreographed and premiered in England in 1936, and in 1940 was acquired by ABT (then called Ballet Theatre) for its first season. The ballet takes place in a garden at a farewell party where a young woman, Caroline, will see her lover one last time before she enters into a marriage of convenience. Her future husband and his former mistress are also at the party. So simple a plot, and yet *Jardin aux Lilas* is one of the most complex ballets ever choreographed—a pas de quatre inside a panorama.

The pictorial plane of Tudor's stage is like no one else's and reflects his turn-of-the-century sensibility, his roots in Edwardian England, when life still seemed to flow by horizontally (it was flowing toward a trench). Like Alfred Tennyson, an earlier A. T., Tudor is a poet of loss—lost love, lost idealism, sometimes lost life—and he uses his corps like lines in a slow-rolling ballad, sending dancers across the stage in unison, their port de bras a curving rhyme of alignment. And he sends them across in waves, so they suggest the sweep, the passage, of time. (From Tennyson's "In Memoriam": "Our little systems have their day;/ They have their day and cease to be:/ They are but broken lights of thee,/ And thou, O Lord, art more than they.")

Against this pictorial flow, four fates rise and fall in high relief. Tudor moves the four leads upstage and down, perpendicular to the

Two Princes and a Mock Tudor

panorama, releasing them into another dimension. He also gives them intimacy, immediacy, by stopping them in tableaux—an embrace, a reach, a rest—friezes of emotion. This is melodrama, not unlike the party in *Now, Voyager* (1942) where Bette Davis and Paul Henreid are webbed across the room by glances only. The four dancers must project this kind of drama, but with their bodies, their backs. Tudor helps them by keeping their port de bras low. Battement, jeté, *sissonne*—these explosive moves are performed with arms down at the sides, hands below shoulders and often below waists. Tudor suggests the straitlaced decorum of the time, the stillness and quiet eloquence of the bust, shoulders, head. "He didn't want the arms to distract," the ballerina Melissa Hayden, who learned the ballet from Tudor, told me after one performance this season. If the arms are down, the dancers must lift and lead with their hearts, which takes a pliant spine, and strength, push, through the pelvis.

Tudor cannot be tossed off. In this way he is different from Balanchine, who loved to see dancers fly, shooting from the hip. As Hayden said, "Tudor is like a painting." She meant the lines had to be where Tudor put them, the dancers in sync musically and spatially, rehearsed to the nth degree. At the same time—like Balanchine—Tudor wanted large-scale performance from his dancers, bodies passionate in space, covering ground. "You have to dance Tudor full out," his former assistant Airi Hynninen told *Ballet Review* in 1995. "When an arabesque droops, so does the spirit."

I saw three of the season's performances of *Jardin*, one in the first week, one midseason, and a matinee at season's end. It was as if ABT was rehearsing the ballet onstage. The first performance was shocking for its lack of cohesion, its droopiness and dropped details (Caroline's distinct good-bye to each guest, for instance). The second performance was better—clearer but still wan. By the last performance, the lines were holding, it was *Jardin aux Lilas*, taut and teeming with details, the stillnesses more powerful, the music, Chausson's *Poème*, sounding newly minted (Tudor's sensory genius is such that his compositional clarity seems to crystallize the music, don't ask me how). This last was the performance

Melissa Hayden saw, and she judged it a dishonor to Tudor: it was still too messy, and the dancing, and consequently the emotions, too small. But I was thankful for the improvement, moved by the "little system" that did come through, and more than ever baffled as to how ABT could treat this heart-stopping ballet—sixty years in its repertory—like secondhand goods.

September 2000

Taylor's Domain

A dancer in Paul Taylor's company is not a bona fide Paul Taylor dancer until he or she develops a particular curve within a phrase. You see it most readily when the dancer runs in a circle in those little scuffing-slipper steps of which Taylor is so fond—the way the entire body is magnetically flexed to the center, the spine answering that empty space, the chin and shoulder listening. Taylor dancers run and jump, walk and crawl, jerk and twitch. But they are never more Taylor dancers than when they move in circles, even if they are circling in one spot on the stage. It is in circles and rings and centrifugal swings that we see them for what they are: forces of nature.

And yet Taylor dancers don't pirouette. Oh, scour the repertory and you might find some. These would be exceptions that prove the rule. The pirouette of classical dance takes place on pointe or demi-pointe, and is an act of high artifice, generally a three-step structure consisting of (1) a preparation in plié, much like a deep breath; (2) up on tiptoe and twirl—the final swirls of a Dairy Queen cone or the coloratura's most difficult trill; (3) down and repose, to show you didn't fall. Taylor has no interest in preparations, and he likes falls. His incomparable *Esplanade* contains a pelting summer storm of flying falls. As for the pirouette, it is something no animal would ever do, and therefore Taylor dancers don't do them either. It's too superego, though he might say prissy or stuffy.

Taylor spent his formative years in the dances of Martha Graham, a mythic realm where superego is constantly grabbed at the heel and pulled down, undermined by id. Dancing with Graham in the 1950s, Taylor knew the fight firsthand, for it is worked into the

Graham technique where a dancer's bright breastbone, his or her angelic liftedness, is constantly undercut, halved and jackknifed in Graham contractions, hungers of the gut and groin. Martha Graham was Modern Dance, the opposite of Ballet. She dragged dance barefoot into a big empty box of sanctified space, then filled it with totems and taboos, mysteries of the couch post-Freud and mid-Jung. Still, Victorian-born, circa 1895, she never let go that golden thread to Heaven.

Taylor severed the thread. Not for him Graham's ancient oracles and high-priestess pronouncements which assumed, by extension, the divinity of man. "I believe in Darwin," he told the *New York Times* in 2001, "and the natural world." And so the tracks and grooves of Taylor technique grow out of the grounded muscularity, the insular physics, of the animal kingdom: the racehorse's heavy tilt into the turn; the big cat's jazzy, deep-shouldered directional shifts within the chase; the concentrated stillness of both prey and predator; the elegant grazing on grasses. Taylor dancers are always Homo sapiens— descended from the apes—human animals rather than human beings. This is a profound distinction.

And it is uniquely Taylor's. Even if he didn't spell it out every once in a while in works like *Three Epitaphs*, where black-masked dancers droop and stoop like the primordial ooze they crawled out of, or *Cloven Kingdom*, which quotes Spinoza in the program note, "Man is a social animal," and sees four men in tails (evening clothes, not fur) performing a series of chest-beating tribal rites, the Taylor dancer embodies this distinction in his or her musculature: strong calves, solid rear, compact and seamless upper body, and again, that flex and curve within a phrase, as if these dancers were bred for leverage, a bipedal torque and balance that lets them roar within the radius of their own limbs, not needing to transcend their bodies as ballet dancers aspire to do (ballet dancers in Taylor are like helium balloons tied to a rail, tugging toward the sky). When the eight o'clock curtain comes up on a Paul Taylor program, it is a thrill distinct from any other in dance. These breathing creatures braced before us, they may not have moved a muscle but the energy is already flying. And if it's just men onstage, as in *Cascade*, one of this season's program openers, the thrill doubles, because Taylor men, even those who ride a fine line of chubbiness, are magnificent—the NFL and Michelangelo's *David*, Man o' War and Mister Ed, all rolled up into one.

Taylor has a New York season once a year, and in that season he usually presents two new works. He likes introducing new works in twos, and there is often an obvious duality in what he's done, one dance savage, the other soft, or maybe acid and ice cream, cutting edge and elegy, sci-fi and slapstick (this March it was *Fiends Angelical* and *Dandelion Wine*, sinister and sunny). This game of oppositions is yet another pitch and curve within the repertory, as if Taylor is saying he's not subject to any one theatrical tradition or temperament, not placing one ideal above another. Taylor isn't in thrall to any ideal, to any dogma beyond Darwin's: objective observance of the natural world. What he sees is what we get. And he sees like a collector—in genus, in genres, in populations, and in pools.

This makes great sense for a dance company, which is tribal after all, and it's one of the reasons Taylor has enjoyed such longevity: he never runs out of subjects or specimens. It's also a reason Taylor gets attacked every few years by critics who want more "adult sexuality" on his stage, another way of saying they want more conventional male-female partnering—the R-rated repartee of movies or the only-you romanticism of Balanchine (in other words, they're not getting their quota of vicarious thrill, i.e., self-projection into the clinches). Taylor isn't concerned with the genital stirrings of character A for character B; he's more interested in the group pheromone, as in his megahit of 1992, *Company B*, in which erotic energies are heightened, enlarged, by WWII and the threat of premature death. Taylor's most recent masterpiece, *Piazzolla Caldera*, really is R-rated, a rite of spring wearing the black lace of the bull ring, wielding a sharp tango heel, and complete with sacrificial maiden—a girl who's sort of slutty. But again, the soloists who momently come forward in their own dank spotlight, showing us their ache or itch, are always step-locked back into the whole, the bristling backroom pool of vice and desire, where they take their place in the pattern, linked up in the eternal circle.

This locking device of Taylor's is yet another aspect of the compleat

Paul Taylor dancer. When they want to they can end a phrase like a gong, striking stillness with such energy that you see a bit of kick-back, a vibration that anchors the image. As with the full-body curve, not all Taylor dancers lock in with the same weight and impact. It tends to be senior dancers, especially senior men, who achieve this level of virtuosity. And it may be a prerequisite to ascent within the company. The amazing Andrew Asnes, with his lush musculature almost laughably perfect and a happy hunger to do it all bigger, faster, cleaner—he could ring like a bell. When Asnes left the company last year, the gleaming Patrick Corbin slid effortlessly into seniority, more understated, stylized, his crew-cut centurion's profile a portrait in helmeted concentration and strength. Corbin's performances aren't introverted, but to some extent he is. As the critic Joel Lobenthal observed, "He comes onstage with a concept," which means he's not go-with-the-flow, he is the flow. Corbin's presence in a dance is like the vibrant hum of a tuning fork, a subliminal wave in the atmosphere. He's the most elegant male dancer in America. And when he's unsubtle, he's that much funnier. In *Company B*, as geeky Johnny the girls can't get enough of ("You're not handsome it's true/but when I look at you/Johnny oh Johnny oh Johnny oh"), when Corbin pushes his chess-champ glasses back up his nose he bucks his head as if swallowing a pill—all on the dotted note. You wonder, where's the Adam's apple? The spaz timing is sublime.

But this is yet another level on which Taylor works, the way he's willing to amplify his own compositional tactics and tics for an air-quote, cartoon quality. In *Funny Papers*, a throwaway dance from 1994 that looks larger and wittier with every passing year (it was only this season I noticed the spoof of Merce Cunningham that sits near the start), the lock effect is like the heavy outline in a comic strip. In 1999's *Oh, You Kid!*, the company's senior female, Lisa Viola, has a sideshow solo that fuses Bloody Mary from *South Pacific* with Dainty June from *Gypsy*. A tour de force for Viola, it's one of the weirdest solos Taylor has ever devised, a string of vaudeville kicks and tricks, with poses so heavily punctuated they read like deadpan double takes. The whole thing is reverb.

Perhaps the deepest reverberation in Taylor is one that is

unconscious. In 1980 Taylor paid brilliant homage to Vaslav Nijinsky's *Le Sacre du Printemps*, that grand spasm of 1913, the first aesthetic breakaway of the twentieth century. Taylor's own *Le Sacre du Printemps (The Rehearsal)* uses the two-piano reduction of Stravinsky's score, thus creating a black-and-white tonality perfect for his cinematic take on the subject: Taylor's *Sacre* is Hollywood noir, a two-reel ritual, comic and tragic. Still, in his autobiography, *Private Domain*, Taylor mentions Nijinsky only once, noting that in college he read a biography of the dancer-choreographer and found it "fascinating." It is the place of Nijinsky in dance history—a dark, heavy hinge—that sounds in Taylor repertory like an echo from the depths, a kind of unbidden muscle memory.

"I am a man and not a beast . . . I am a man and not God . . . I am the earth." Nijinsky's struggle to understand what he was, what the life of the body is meant to be, plays out in his diaries—madly imaginative or just plain mad depending on one's tolerance for poetic obsession splintering into nonsense. The same struggle, however, found a pagan formality in Nijinsky's dances. In *L'Après-midi d'un Faune*, his nymphs and faun (which he danced) are stylized sideways, moving in a kind of bas relief that grounds them. Tight twists at the waist accentuate the feral tension between two and three dimensions, between Debussy's throbbing swirl of sound and physiques so flattened they might be slipping between senses (Mallarmé's poem lies somewhere between memory and dream). In *Sacre* a year later, Nijinsky's stooped and circling peasants curl their hands in at the wrists, little fists of introversion, blunt and mute. Their hands and feet have become clubs and hooves with which they beat out ritual time on hard ground, setting the stage for sacrifice, a girl's death for the good of the crops—"I am the earth." At their premieres, shortly before the stroke of WWI, these dances were considered blasphemous. Even today, ninety years later, they remain symbols hot to the touch, intense metaphors for a sudden internal plunge, an inarticulate, irrevocable shift in the mind-body balance.

Taylor's *Sacre* was not part of the programming this season, but his *Arabesque* was. When it premiered in 1999, I dismissed the dance as not up to much, a little stop-start, and tonally odd (the use of Debussy in a bare-chested temple dance). This year, though, it shone like aged ivory, and its rhythms had the jump and flicker of a candle flame. A note in the program calls *Arabesque* "an ornate pattern with reflected figures," and if the dance had a set, it might be a shadowy mihrab carved and niched with Islamic arabesques. But the "reflected figure" is not just the arabesque. Santo Loquasto's costumes nod to a Diaghilev-era exoticism, the Ballets Russes of *Schéhérazade* and *Le Dieu Bleu*, ballets in which Nijinsky starred. Moreover, it was the music of Debussy that Nijinsky used in two of his three iconoclastic ballets. And the dancers' hands, they're curled in that little *Sacre* club fist. Taylor's reflected figure is Nijinsky, and, thinking back over the Taylor repertory, one begins to feel that Nijinsky's footprint may have left a more pungent impression than Graham's (for all her talk about the ground, Graham's bare foot is never dirty). So much swarm and sacrifice in the dances of Paul Taylor, the call of the wild by moonlight and altar light. And so often a use of the body in profile, faunlike, with that twist at the waist to show the animal is man. Indeed, Nijinsky's famously thick-legged, round-muscled physique is pure Taylor. At the same time: critical distance, peace with man's place in the food chain, an ease and strength within the skin. Maybe this is why audiences leave Taylor in such high spirits. Even at extremes, he's just so balanced.

The program that began with *Arabesque* closed with *Musical Offering*, a dance first performed in 1986. It was an achievement then, a high-water mark both choreographically and in terms of execution. Because dancing is so grueling (especially dancing Taylor) and the career of a dancer so short, companies continually blossom and drop over the years, depending on how many within the company are hitting and holding their stride, how many are past prime or not yet there. Taylor's company right now, except for Corbin, Viola, Kristi Egtvedt, and Richard Chen See, is in an immature phase (with Michael Trusnovec coming on like an engine). When Taylor joined the dancers in their curtain call after *Musical Offering*, he gave them a thumbs up, a gesture I've never seen him make before, as if to say, You got through. But the company in the mid to late eighties was flush, shoulder-deep in compleat Paul Taylor dancers. And *Musical Offering*—a dance built out of circles and curls, ringing stops and stillnesses struck in stone—seemed to rise up like a monument to the company's palpable, physical coherence. It is a dance that Taylor calls "a requiem." But for what? The short life of the dancer? The cyclic rise and fall of the company?

It is set to Anton Webern's orchestration of Bach's sixteen-part exploration of one theme, which is its own circling monument to Baroque musical structure. Leave it to Taylor to hear in this steeple of sound the crying voice of an ancient culture. But listen to the theme; it does seem to blow down over a mountain path. And the dancers respond to it with awe and obedience. Taylor sees them as primitive figures, girded in leather loincloths and headbands. He locks them into a language of totemic poses and strange slow-motion leitmotifs: they beat their chests with little fists in a dream trance, making X's over their hearts; they raise their palms, upper body planted back in submission to the sky. And throughout the piece, like a metronome, they rock sideways on stiff legs, another X, as if they are imitating their own statues of worship. These big, simple shapes, keening and mourning, fit into a circulatory system of rounds and whirlpools, stately processions and pietà poses, and soon the dance is just pouring out as from a heavy urn, all its evocations—Bach's everlasting command, Nijinsky's inchoate ritual, the body's mortal matter—joined in one current. It is a long dance, and yet it is never long enough, so sustained is the tone of stoicism, so inventive this vision of wordless lament pouring into emptiness, the salt and the sand. Animals die, Taylor seems to say, but what powerful imprints we leave behind.

May 2001

Petipaw

In his New York apartment, George Balanchine had an Audubon print of a bald eagle. It was in his living room; you can see it in the famous photographs of Balanchine playing with his cat Mourka. In these photos the cat is in the air, fully stretched yet twisting in the middle, utterly rapt yet strangely relaxed, not unlike Fred Astaire snapped between steps. Balanchine is often crouched lower than the cat, urging it on, as if coaching a dancer in a complicated jeté *en tournant*. Behind them, perched in profile, is the eagle. It is a wonderful trio—cat, raptor, choreographer—all three evolved in the same direction, with the same physiological assets: sharp eyes that miss nothing, traplike claws for catching life, and senses attuned to sound, smell, movement, gesture. For these three creatures, seeing and hearing are kinetic acts, a wiring beneath and beyond thought.

Balanchine died in 1983, but even when he was alive it seemed unfair to measure other choreographers against him. Frederick Ashton and Antony Tudor were great artists (the influence of Tudor's early *Jardin aux Lilas* on Balanchine's late *Davidsbündlertänze* is a provocative bit of shadow play, a nod of homage better late than never). But in the sheer breadth and amplitude of Balanchine's gifts, even these geniuses were brought down a notch. To hold Balanchine as a point of comparison for today's choreographers is still more and rather wildly unfair. Gens X, Y, and Z have loads (or maybe I should say, downloads) of information, but no experience of the wide world their predecessors knew (Kerouac's "road" is now Microsoft's "highway"). And yet, what can we do? There is no escaping Balanchine as a standard. The deep and palpable dimensionality of his ballets, that sense of invisible architecture popping up before our eyes, of landscapes teeming with growing, breathing things—in short, his glorious, continuous exploration of what a ballet can be and do—all this seems lost on youngsters making their first, second, and third works for New York City Ballet and American Ballet Theatre. In the last few years, ballets premiered at these companies have been so flat and faceless and monotonal and dimensionless that the word *premiere* has begun to seem more punishment than promise.

The late critic David Daniel, when he could be dragged to the theater to see something new (or was told over the phone about a recent dubious effort), loved to purr ominously, "It's the end of civilization as we know it." Pushed for analysis, he fixed on the television screen as the great reductive force in American culture. There it was, shaped like a stage—a box—but without any depth or life, in fact, a vacuum. It was insanely quixotic, commercial breaks every five minutes. And most damaging, instead of being larger than life, scaled for wonder, it was very much smaller. To the teat of television, we can add the quick addictions of the computer—video games, the internet, virtual this and that. The extreme sports that a tiny minority of Americans engage in (and the rest watch on TV) are the antidotal flip side to the extreme slouch of the couch potato and the computer junkie, sedentary sensibilities happy to gaze (or glaze) upon a depthless screen making synthetic sounds. As my best friend with two sons says, "It's a battle to keep your kids in three dimensions." The same with ballet.

Case in point. In January, NYCB presented a new work by company corps member Melissa Barak. It was a piece called *Telemann Overture Suite in E Minor*, and Barak made it for the School of American Ballet's 2001 workshop performance. The ballet impressed NYCB director Peter Martins, and he asked Barak to set it on the company. But what was it that impressed him? Barak's work possesses a youthful bounciness that no doubt looked good on the students at SAB, and she keeps the bodies moving. But keeping the bodies moving isn't enough. It isn't even the point. What about relationships, flirtations, competitions, quests? Barak's dancers are like smiling members of a commune, so equal they flatline in friendliness. What about Telemann? The atmosphere of the baroque, the theater of his day, the dance forms of his time? A reference to any of these might have opened out, or dramatically enlarged, the ballet. Instead, it all takes place on one level, ground level, as if the stage were an empty lot before the building goes up. For the twenty minutes of *Telemann*, amid rows of romps and kicks, nothing happens.

It was pretty hard on Barak that her ballet shared the program with two little Balanchines, *Monumentum Pro Gesualdo* (1960) and *Movements for Piano and Orchestra* (1963). They're both short and spare, so short they've been teamed up in the repertory. Even together they can seem slight, nothing really. And yet, everything. *Monumentum* is set to madrigals by Don Carlo Gesualdo, which Stravinsky recomposed for orchestra; *Movements*, also by Stravinsky, uses serial technique. So both scores are planted in a time. Balanchine uses that. His *Monumentum* is grave and lyric, with a recurring pattern of narrow diagonals like long corridors. There's a cathedral feeling of vaults and stained-glass windows. And the tender pawing motion of the women's legs, they might be unicorns wrought, pictured, in those windows. The ballet's famous series of tosses—ballerina in arabesque, thrown high into the arms of partners—feels like white doves loosed at the altar. *Movements*, which follows after a pause, has none of the old-stone reverberation of *Monumentum*. Its silences and stillnesses are aggressive, the abyss that lives in every laboratory. Stravinsky described the women in *Movements* as "a hexachord of those beelike little girls who seem to be bred to the eminent choreographer's specifications." They do look bred in test tubes. They could be dangerous.

These Balanchine "nothings"—so rich in natural phenomena, the imagery of the spire and the scientist, and so plainly invoking two types of faith—to see them next to the latest offerings is to be struck by how denatured most new ballets are, how empty they are of beating hearts (other than the aerobic kind) and various levels of movement. But then, there's no nature in a computer screen. No outdoors or weather, ditches and rises, the sudden flush of other life. And even if young choreographers aren't online, do they understand that they have to let go of the barre and see the world? Even if it's only watching pigeons in Central Park?

I remember the late 1980s, when Paul Taylor and Merce Cunningham were carrying the day, growing greater as they would have anyway, but in the context of Balanchine's death their power doubly profound. Look, their new work seemed to say, there is still genius here. I remember a conversation between a balletomane, another critic, and me. The 'mane referred to Merce Cunningham's dances as "ballets." The critic took issue with that. Cunningham was postmodern; his whole ethos was a reaction against the expectations of classical dance; to call his dances ballets was a contradiction in terms, willfully naive. The conversation made an impression because both were right. Still, I couldn't help siding with the 'mane. Cunningham may have made philosophical choices that had aesthetic ramifications, but he was born to a world saturated with classicism and came of age during civilization as we knew it, the old taxonomies intact.

In recent years, when Cunningham became too physically impaired to move around the studio, he began using a computer program called Lifeforms, mapping his dances with a click and slide. And yet his work never lost its creaturely feel, its prickly skin and warm-bloodedness. In a recent *American Masters* documentary on Cunningham, one of the surprises was his morning ritual. Cunningham sketches daily—pictures of birds, mostly shorebirds, and with an acute eye for the character of a species as revealed through posture and grouping. Like Balanchine, the predator's eye for life and form. From these delightful and true sketches, the camera cut to a tape of Cunningham's *Beach Birds* from 1991. We're not supposed to say that Cunningham's dances are "about" anything, but given the title, and the dancers wearing unitards halved in black and white, an evocation of laughing gulls was clearly at hand. The dance plays with the seemingly empty patience with which these birds stand on the beach, the sort of *I Ching* toss of their groupings, the random landings and liftoffs. As only the cry of a gull in the air can do, the dance questions the meaning of life, the transience, the wind that blows the sand. It is nothing and everything, beneath and beyond, gulls there but not there. Look at a work like *Beach Birds* and you begin to understand that the absence of dimension in our new ballets is an absence of metaphor and simile, the time-honored tools of the poet. Great choreography *is* poetry, and where would poetry be without its nightingales and glowworms and long-legged flies and fleas, without the leaps and flights they bring the artist. Wallace Stevens: "I know noble accents/And lucid, inescapable rhythms;/ But I know, too,/ That the blackbird is involved/ In what I know."

Classical ballet of the nineteenth century is a Noah's ark of nature and a primer in the job of making metaphors and similes. One need only look to that cornerstone of dance classicism, *The Sleeping Beauty*, to see a garlanded hierarchy of court creatures: mice, rats, cats, birds, wolves, and the implied horses and hounds of the Hunt Scene. Even in the Act Three wedding, when God's in his heaven and the natural and supernatural worlds are joined, creatures run true to form. In the Bluebird pas de deux, for instance, scholars have puzzled over Princess Florine's signature gesture—hand to ear, as if hearing a whisper. Was this movement merely coquettish or did it mean something? I've never forgotten the answer of an aging ballerina on a dance panel: Florine is like a bird, the woman said, she's listening and wary because she hears Puss 'n Boots, a cat, in the wings.

Trained at Russia's Mariinsky Theatre, Balanchine learned all its lessons. The swan queens and white cats and bluebirds live on in his ballets as echoes, intonations, and sighs, leitmotivs that sing to the music, transmuting space into place (when the port de bras of Odette is worked into the ballerina role in "Diamonds," you feel the water of the lakeside has frozen into an ice-crystal palace). But Balanchine didn't limit himself to what he inherited from Petipa, Ivanov, and the rest. His ballets brim with his own observations, things animal, vegetable, and mineral, beginning with the Siren in *The Prodigal Son*: she's a black widow spider in a red hourglass chiton. Think of the chambered nautilus in *Concerto Barocco*—an inner ear hearing Bach hearing God creating life. *The Four Temperaments*, choreographed and premiered on the shallow stage of the High School of Needle Trades, is full of shape-shifting, morphing form—stinging insects and stony sphinxes and even a small cyclone. As if to show how imaginative energy can implode and open even the flattest strip of space, in *4Ts* Balanchine turns a sidewalk of stage into a Nile of the mind (this is why Balanchine never needed elaborate sets—"place" was created in the floor pattern and the steps). And then there's the greenery winding through the entire repertory, daisy chains and garlands and girls with weeping willow hair, all climbing and stemming from one root, the tree with the apple that opened our eyes.

The clearest, and dearest, example of what I'm talking about is in *Apollo*. Made in 1928, it is Balanchine's coming-of-age ballet, and young Apollo, learning how to use his power, is very much the young choreographer himself. Apollo has three muses whom he puts through their paces and learns from in return. The four are playmates, but the idyll cannot last. Late in the ballet, the muses seat themselves on the floor, each with a leg extended forward so their three points touch and their legs are like three rays of light, a small bonfire. As Apollo walks around them they follow him with their eyes, and when he's behind them they keep him in view by dropping their heads back, the way cats do, in a gaze that follows full circle. It's a kind of limbic attention outside human nature; anyone who has lived with cats has seen them do this, follow the same movement in unblinking synchronicity. It is cozy too, three kittens on a hearth, and elemental, the spell of the sun upon the earth. Pulling from his system what he'd seen of cats, Balanchine gives us a phenomenon, the muses' silent understanding that Apollo has changed, he's ready to be a god. When Balanchine told friends, as reported in Bernard Taper's 1984 biography, *Balanchine*, that he wanted to present Mourka in a public program titled "The Evolution of Ballet: From Petipa to Petipaw," he was, in a way, describing what he'd been doing all along.

Last year, New York City Ballet created a new position, Resident Choreographer, for Christopher Wheeldon. A NYCB soloist, formerly of England's Royal Ballet, Wheeldon had been making ballets since his teens and he was ready to make them full time. So he stopped dancing, which was a loss; his presence onstage was 110 percent. To see him as the happy lover in *A Midsummer Night's Dream*, picking imaginary flowers oh so preciously (like an eager decorator matching swatches), was to glimpse the John Gielguds and Benny Hills in every Englishman's background. Still, Wheeldon brings his 110 percent to his own ballets. It's clear he adores the art, which is more than you can say for a lot of classical choreographers these days.

You can see that Wheeldon wants to make ballets that are places in time and space. He wants those deep dimensions, those golden keys to other realms. He has easy musicality and a big natural gift for making lovely and unexpected *enchaînements*. And yet in ballet after promising ballet, Wheeldon seems to hit up against his ambitions, as if the lock won't turn. In his collaborations with the set designer Ian Falconer, Wheeldon has actually imposed dimension upon the ballets through odd angles and extreme strategies of staging. Because of this—and I admire his reach—the ballets tend to begin better than they end. Wheeldon's *enchaînements* are so immediately disarming that it takes some time to see he hasn't animated the ballet from the inside—he's not working metaphorically. *Scènes de Ballet*, a piece Wheeldon choreographed on SAB students, opens breathtakingly, the stage split with a barre slanting down the middle. The students on one side are reality. The students on the other side are a mirror reflection—another dimension! What a wonderful point of departure. But as this classroom ballet progresses from barre to center to a pas de deux for an older boy and girl, it loses that twilight-zone strangeness, that displacement unique to dancers, so much of their lives lived in a mirror. The fantasy doesn't climax or burst or dissolve interestingly. It just sort of goes away. Jerome Robbins saw this same dancer-and-mirror duality as an atmospheric intoxication. He turned his dancers into dream creatures, the faun and nymph of Mallarmé's *L'Après-midi d'un Faune*, set to music by Debussy. This gave him a whole other order of movement from which to draw— feral sensuality, animal languor. Other orders of movement, this is what Wheeldon must learn to use.

He comes closer in his hit from last season, *Polyphonia*. Set to ten piano pieces—oddball, exploratory, droll—by Gyorgy Ligeti, the ballet is a distillation of several choreographic voices (Balanchine, Robbins, Martins). It is precise and witty, an accomplished pastiche, and it contains a tender shoot of metaphor, the second duet, which is danced by Wendy Whelan and Jock Soto. Mysterious, amphibious, she's like a deep-sea creature, opening and closing, floating up and around Soto. This duet feels like the heart of the ballet, but it comes too early to act as a culmination or as the answer to a question. Indeed, Whelan's rarely-touching-the-ground sinuousness is in whispering dialogue with Allegra Kent's floating phantom in Balanchine's *Ivesiana*, "The Unanswered Question" section. Wheeldon has created his own unanswered question: Where are we, what is she? Even though the music is Ligeti, I kept thinking of Saint-Saëns's *Carnival of the Animals*—"Aquarium." When Whelan and Soto come back in Part Nine, they bring their enclosed flow with them and the audience leans in. We've seen something happening. The ballet ends as it begins, with the dancers' Machine Age shadows cast huge upon the cyclorama. *Polyphonia* is a bit too slick to be satisfying, but that little pocket of life stays with you.

Variations Sérieuses is both a step back, to something more concrete, and a step forward, it brims. It is a comic ballet about a ballet company, set literally onstage. Falconer's clever set puts the audience in the wings, stage left. Talk about dimension. It's a view on a ballet I've never seen before. With charm and economy, Wheeldon brings on the characters—the ballerina, the premier danseur, the young girl, the ballet master, the corps—and tells his backstage story, which is basically *All About Eve* in toe shoes. Because Wheeldon is so focused on getting this world right and doing it in a way that gives pleasure, he reaches in all the right directions. When the diva ballerina gets angry she paws the ground like a snorting bull. Corps girls flutter and peck like hens. There's a barnyard brio to company life, and the young girl in her white leotard is like something just emerged, translucent, from the chrysalis in the eaves. She's the connection between backstage and onstage, for the ballet she understudies is about sylphs—the tutus have little wings.

The pragmatism required by such storytelling is liberating for Wheeldon. (I have long felt it would help young choreographers if they were given stiffer assignments or pointed exercises, like the kinds one used to get in acting classes: pretend you're a lettuce in love; make a pas de deux for porcupines.) Wheeldon lays in all kinds of details and observations, making references (there's an Astaire-inspired dance for four stagehands with brooms) and allusions: the young girl's opening solo is full of turns in attitude, the pose of Mercury and a forecast of her mercurial rise. The ballet is booming with life.

When *Variations Serieuses* was premiered last spring, the ending was weak (to be honest, I can't remember how it ended). But Wheeldon has fixed the ending. Now, as in *Polyphonia*, he brings the ballet around full circle. His next choreographic challenge is to make an ending that doesn't circle back, that is instead a surprise even to itself. Here, however, the ending works. The young girl—a diva now, flouncing and pouting like the one before her—watches another spidery corps girl tiptoe onto the empty stage, just as she once had, hungry for stardom. It's the eternal Eve Harrington—there's always one in the wings—and a nice nip of an ending, a sting of recognition. Paradise and predators, feathers and claws. What is ballet but two genres in one body? Metaphysical poetry and melodrama.

March 2002

How Good Is the Kirov?

The Kirov Ballet is the company George Balanchine left behind when he sailed from Russia in 1924. It is the company from which Rudolf Nureyev defected in 1961, followed by Natalia Makarova in 1970 and Mikhail Baryshnikov in 1974. Formerly known as the Imperial Ballet of the Mariinsky Theatre (named after Czar Alexander II's wife, Marie), the Kirov is the great Russian mother company, a matryoshka doll hatching dancer after dancer—an infinity of dancers—from its Imperial School on Theatre Street, a continuum of star pupils that includes the legendary names Anna Pavlova, Tamara Karsavina, Vaslav Nijinsky. The company that is today called The Kirov Ballet of the Mariinsky Theatre—still Dickensian in its selection standards; still trained within the meticulous, luminous rounds of Vaganova technique; still a constellation of coaches pushing, pulling their protegés to the top—she is always there, like Everest.

But we all have issues with our mothers. Perhaps no ballet company in the world is more daunting to write about than the Kirov. The company has a deep and detailed past which is the stuff of scholars, and a performance history that is hard to know given restrictions during the Cold War. And then there are the politics: the fact that Russian defectors escaped to the United States to dance; that it was Manhattan Balanchine chose as the concrete-and-steel setting for his New York City Ballet; and that it was American dancers on which he built his neoclassical style. Yes, Balanchine cherished his years in the Mariinsky school, drawing deeply on the sights and sounds of his childhood, his Proustian connection to ballets scaled for a czar. Solomon Volkov's book *Balanchine's Tchaikovsky*, a series of interviews in which the choreographer talks about the composer, is a rich remembrance of things past in St. Petersburg ("Everyone thinks the tsar's box at the Mariinsky Theatre is in the middle. But actually, it was on the side, on the right. . . . We would be lined up by size and presented. We were given chocolate in silver boxes, wonderful ones!"). Once Balanchine got down to work in America, however, he had to use what was at hand—no czars, no state school housing a classical tradition, no old-world chocolates, but instead, strong, long-boned, USDA bodies ready to work hard to be classical. Balanchine had to start from scratch, and he began by establishing his School of American Ballet. Necessity would be the mother of invention.

What does this mean in practical terms? That Balanchine would choreograph to American strengths: a leggy athleticism, a competitive desire to prove oneself, a direct and down-to-earth presentation. He sought that quality of the quotidian that all mid-century American moderns were seeing as higher truth. "'Don't pretend to dance,' he would say," writes Suki Schorer in the first chapter of her recent book *Balanchine Technique*. It was another way of saying, don't pretend to be what you are not, dancers with a deep tradition. New York was a new world and this was a classicism dimensionally unmoored, thinner, more linear, more musically prodigal—not Genesis, but Revelations—a powerful next chapter in the history of classical dance.

Balanchine believed in both God and fate, and it is in keeping with the mystic aspect of his life that after leaving Russia and landing in Diaghilev's Ballets Russes he choreographed *The Prodigal Son* (1929), a dance with an angular, openly sexual pas de deux between a rebellious boy and a looming, elusive Siren, Felia Doubrovska of the long long legs. But Balanchine never did go home. He continued to heed the siren's song, and forever following that song, he made a repertory in the West that is its own world with its own metaphysics. In short, the prodigal climbed to messiah status, and in the last year of his life, when his *Catalogue of Works* was finally published, he kept it at his bedside where it was referred to as "the Bible." When the Kirov comes to New York, it's a bit like the Old Testament abutting the New—a defensive sense of competing religions creeps into people's responses.

How Good Is the Kirov?

The catechism began in 1989, when, after a twenty-five-year absence and in the spirit of glasnost, the Kirov Ballet came to New York's Metropolitan Opera House with two Balanchine ballets included in its repertory—*Theme and Variations* and *Scotch Symphony*. There was much coverage of the event, emotions focusing on what a great step into the present tense it was for the Russians, and how poignant it would be to see Balanchine danced by the company of his upbringing. And it *was* poignant. But there was also a general feeling of uncertainty, a discomfited jostling over what the Kirov should be striving for in its dancing of Balanchine. There were those who wanted a City Ballet facsimile, who seemed to feel the Kirov was old-fashioned and outmoded and should just Go West. Why aren't the dancers rolling through the foot like we do? Why aren't they faster, more forward in the hips? Why? For the same reason our dancers don't have the Kirov's majesty in stillness, or the upper-body energy to carry a fairy tale, a century, in their arms. It's not what either is trained to do. For those who excused the Kirov's not being NYCB there was magic in the company's *Theme and Variations*, in the tonal connection between *Theme* and the company's full-length *Sleeping Beauty* (also performed that tour)—a lullaby weight that makes the court palpable, a sense of forever that breathes in the bourrées.

At the time, the Kirov was run by Oleg Vinogradov, and the roster of ballerinas was a mixed bag. There were older women of great integrity like Tatiana Terekhova and Galina Mezentseva, but they were deemed Soviet in style and thus passé. Altynai Asylmuratova was the chosen one, having been earlier anointed in *The New Yorker*. She had a dark ardor, a Tartar princess face, but a faulty technique which she hid under excesses of line and a puffed-up posture. Yulia Makhalina was coming up fast, yet she too reached for extremes of line, her dancing as overdone, labored, as little Zhanna Ayupova's was modest, light. The funny thing is, the afterimages I hold from that engagement, the moments burned in memory, belong to the two women least poised to please on American terms. I still see blond, plain Terekhova in attitude on pointe, fixed in space as if bronzed; and Mezentseva in *Scotch Symphony*, a wraith in pink tulle, a pinwheeling ghost.

Landscape with Moving Figures

Vinogradov favored the Makhalinas. In the early 1990s, perhaps in the reach to read globally, company style went to new extremes, the principal women becoming too attenuated and too deliberate at once, stretching *and* slowing (the worst of West and East). When the Kirov brought an all-Diaghilev bill to New York in 1995—an evening of Firebirds and Golden Slaves, velvet pillows and beaded bras—the company seemed to be at sea in the exotic, all slinky navels and snaky limbs. That was the season in which Uliana Lopatkina surfaced, with her Theda Bara eyes and body as taut as a tusk. Kirov ballet dancing was beginning to look like Russian ice dancing, a sort of skinny kitsch classicism shipped in for tourists.

But as I've written before in these pages, dance companies wax and wane, fade and blossom. And shortly after that 1995 engagement things changed. Vinogradov, an impassive man who ran the company coldly and unfortunately was getting it to dance that way, was expelled in a financial scandal. After an interim leadership shared by Farukh Ruzimatov and Makhar Vasiev, both Kirov principals at the time, Vasiev was made director of the ballet. And he was answering to Valery Gergiev, the uncompromising conductor who'd been artistic director of the Kirov Opera since 1988, and who in 1996 became director of the entire Mariinsky Theatre, thus bringing a blazing international spotlight to the ballet.

Who can say what is the best recipe for artistic regeneration? Certainly there can be none without raw material in the corps. But there must also be someone driving at the top, a leader with teeth and taste. Having a world-renowned musician at the helm of the Mariinsky has been a compelling development. And Vasiev, who directs the company daily, clearly has an eye for talent, a gift for proportion. When the Kirov returned to the Met in 1999, with a restored version of its original *Sleeping Beauty*, it was as if the company itself had woken from a bad dream. Except for some super-high extensions à la *seconde* (leg up by the ear)—an instance of Kirov women catching an obnoxious Western trend—the dancers looked at ease within their skin. The tempos were bright, the line was clean (so much hyperbole pruned away), and the dancing was big. Doing that *Beauty* seemed to jolt the company, remind it of something it was losing in the whole Western question. Kirov history, its theatrical values, its pride of place and placement—that Vaganova upper body which rounds out of the pelvic bowl to make the torso, head, and arms a sphere of infinite poesy—this was something to embrace.

Indeed, the change in Lopatkina was symbolic. So scary in 1995, with her sinews of steel, she returned softer, warmer. In the second movement of Balanchine's *Symphony in C*, she took quiet possession of the music, putting her strength at the service of phrasing, a performance both remote and refined, queen of the cloud forest. In fact, she outdanced any Americans I've seen in the role since. And it wasn't just Lopatkina. Diana Vishneva was setting a standard for fully articulated dancing, her whole body alive, and younger dancers Daria Pavlenko and Veronika Part were rising like cream. When it was announced a few months later that the Kirov was planning to take on Balanchine's *Jewels*—a ballet exquisitely difficult to cast because it requires five phenomenal women, a tall order these days even at NYCB—it seemed not only perfect timing, but a gauntlet tossed with air kisses.

The Kirov came back to the Met for two weeks in July 2002, with *Jewels* programmed for the last three days of the engagement and a restored *La Bayadère* up front. Petipa's 1877 foray into Orientalism, *La Bayadère* is a story of doomed love between a temple dancer and a warrior—a sort of *Giselle* amid the palms and altars of India. As with *The Sleeping Beauty* three years ago, here was an effort to retrieve the original, to see what it looked like, and to trace one's own bone structure in the face of an ancestor. What the company found in *Beauty* was a colorful, brimming, and bumptious affair—a ballet not distant, misty, at all, as so many productions, including the Kirov's, had since become. What we find with this *La Bayadère*, dated to 1900 and pieced together from archives in Russia and at Harvard, is that it too was laid out with more leisure, pockets of concentrated choreography spaced between gay processionals. It's a different rhythm than we're used to, especially as we head into this new century, where third and sometimes even second intermissions are being dropped from full-length ballets, squeezing the ballets tight between babysitters and train schedules, stressing the pace and distorting the shape. These Kirov restorations remind one that ballet is an art of the eye, and the eye must have its rests. It is a reality

Balanchine learned well. His first full-length hit in America was *The Nutcracker* (1954), and he admitted that the Act One party dances were somewhat dull, prosaic; they were there to set up the imaginative flights of Act Two. In this *La Bayadère* the surprise is the Act Four wedding, and it's a wow. No longer a stumpy remnant of an act no one quite remembers, it is now a vivid ricercar, with all the ballet's narrative and expressive motifs—life and death, prose and poetry, pageant and pas de deux—tightly interwoven, compressed, a fugue state in tutus. There is nothing in ballet quite like it.

But ballet is also an art of the ear. Except for a few haunting melodies, *La Bayadère*'s score by Ludwig Minkus is by-the-yard with only passing coherence (one minute it sounds like Tchaikovsky, the next, Offenbach). The restored score doesn't bring additional aural build to the ballet—the final momentum is all Petipa's—and despite the choreographic mastery of Act Four, one can come away feeling that other of the nips and tucks over time have a sense about them. A tighter *Bayadère* may be a better *Bayadère*. For where *The Sleeping Beauty* makes continuity, life, its theme, thereby benefiting from duration, a horizontal flow, *La Bayadère* is all vows and venom, a triangle between love, murder, and eternity. The distillation that has occurred over the decades, the cutting away of explanatory scenes set to shallow music (as when the ghost of Nikiya appears in Solor's bedroom), makes for steeper narrative drop-offs, a terrain more in tune with this ballet of pitch and abyss.

Just as in *The Sleeping Beauty*, it was inspiring to see these dancers engage with the wide vistas opening around them. When Vladimir Ponomarev, the High Brahmin in red robes, plants himself at the footlights, he might be a baritone braced for his opening note, pulling it up by the root. The dancers have a sense of theater—the spotlight and the gaslight and the stage as a space without a ceiling, larger than life. Some might call this corny, but seeing it anew, art as unshakeable belief, I felt how much I miss it. I think audiences miss it too, which goes a long way to explaining why opera, a high art not nearly as audience-friendly as dance (even *with* supertitles), has the fastest growing following of all the performing arts. *La Bayadère* set the scale for this engagement as well as the standard for dancing, line that sings to an ideal, a line you see even in the men.

I feel sympathy for the male dancer of today. Our taste for superstars, for macho guys who've defected from somewhere or who treat ballet as an artsy form of sport, is a law of diminishing returns. One need only look at the troubling trajectory of Angel Corella at American Ballet Theatre. So promising in his first years—pure raw talent—he seemed to be reaching for artistry, working with focus. But the last three Met seasons have seen him settle for cheap flash, hard sell, a giving-in you see in his physique, which has literally settled (his legs look thicker, his line shorter). Carlos Acosta, another technical wiz, joined ABT this season. He was formerly with the Houston Ballet, where much was made of his having come from Cuba (well, there aren't too many places left to defect from). We seem to need backstory in our men, extracurricular derring-do. And yet the ABT season's most exciting performances from a male dancer came from Marcelo Gomes, a tall, dark, ardent young man whose most exotic bit of biographical data is that he studied with the Paris Opéra Ballet. Gomes dares to care about classicism. He has gorgeous *épaulement* (the nuanced modeling of the upper body)—quite a bit better than most ABT women—and a yearning port de bras. In his debut *Giselle* with Paloma Herrera, the Act Two dancing was so curvaceously wrought, so insular, it seemed they were alone in a bower in a bubble. You could see Herrera respond to this intimacy (who wouldn't?). She found a new softness in herself.

I can't say what will happen to Gomes at ABT, whether he will eventually give way to jock posturing or will be encouraged to follow his lights. But I thought of him while watching the Kirov. "These men are not afraid to be beautiful." It is the first thing I wrote in my notebook, and the first flush of pleasure the company offered: men dancing with whole hearts (not an eye watching the audience watch them), and a refinement that reached to the fingertips. As Solor in *La Bayadère*, Andrian Fadeyev and Viacheslav Samodurov both performed mime that drew up from the tailbone, articulation something between animal and angel, a mammalian largesse. All the men seemed to be working in the grain of their particular gifts. There was Fadeyev's aristocratic dispatch; Samodurov's compact landings, swiftly torqued; Vasili Scherbakov's arrow-like loft and eiderdown aplomb; Danila Korsuntsev's rangy grace. No one was fighting to take the stage by swagger.

As the company moved through its program of *La Bayadère*s, *Don Q*'s, and *Swan Lake*s, heading toward the floating castle that is *Jewels*, its greatest glory was revealed: the ballerinas. There isn't a company in the world as rich in the real thing—Diana Vishneva, Veronika Part, Daria Pavlenko, Zhanna Ayupova, Sofia Gumerova, Irina Golub (never mind that more than half these women are soloists, not principals). Formidable arabesques, beautiful feet, tight fifths, eloquent backs, legs raised and held like broadswords. The women, to a one, are completely pulled up in the spine but with gravity, peace, in the shoulders (no pinching during the difficult parts, no stiff chins). It is an utterly integrated play between reach and roundness that creates this Kirovian aura of atmosphere, a volumetric glamour that's like an invisible stole, the night around the moon. In *Don Quixote*, when Natalia Sologub danced the Queen of the Dryads variation—a big sharp solo that no one can do anymore without jerking adjustments (it's full of swinging fouettés *en tournant* and sudden stops)—her freedom within its winging precision was jaw-dropping. She might have been snapping open large linen napkins, then folding them corner to corner, crisp and neat. The house roared, as if to say, So after all, it can be done.

The Kirov debuted *Jewels* back in 1999 in St. Petersburg, took it to London in 2000, and first performed it in America last February at the Kennedy Center. It's been a winding path to the Big Apple. To see the Russians in this looming Balanchine after nine days of story ballets was to see them with nothing on but their dancing. And what a sight.

Balanchine choreographed *Jewels* in 1967, three years after NYCB moved from City Center to the State Theater at Lincoln Center. It was meant to be a big ballet that would fill the big new stage that was now the company's home. Did Balanchine ever imagine *Jewels* would be danced across the plaza at the Met, on a stage that makes the State Theater's look small? When the curtains opened on that deep, high, wide wash of soft green light, a cascade of gems swirling on the cyclorama as if shaken from a jeweler's pouch in Heaven, I thought, It's like a hole in the universe, a vast outer space. This set was based on the original *Jewels* set, which was later redesigned; the current NYCB set has gems pasted on the cyc like a necklace laid flat. The difference in these sets, glittering riches from on high versus a glowing abstraction, is indicative of the differences in performance. Where City Ballet dances the three sections of *Jewels* ("Emeralds," "Rubies," "Diamonds") as a state of mind, a multifaceted meditation on one theme—the tension between the quest and the capture—the Russians are attuned to fantasy. It's as if they're in a Balanchine theme park, a starry Disneyland romance of Fauré's France, Stravinsky's America, and Tchaikovsky's Russia—panoramas filled with fabled creatures.

It's intoxicating, the Kirov splendor in *Jewels*. Not only did they dance every step, they danced in a way that would have had Balanchine beaming—not because they move like Balanchine dancers (they don't) but because the dancing is so rich and full and listening and large. Veronika Part, voluptuous yet slim, luxuriant yet light, was a kind of milkmaid princess in the second lead of "Emeralds." She filled the stage. In "Rubies," Diana Vishneva shook it up like dice. This is a dancer who can do anything technically, but sometimes gets pulled off course by her own strong will (her Tuesday night *Bayadère* was an unguided missile, white heat, out of control). But "Rubies" is about will, and Vishneva gets it in a big way, treating us to a one-woman Broadway show—*Guys and Firebirds*. Hers was one of those giddy performances in which virtuosity, all cylinders firing, reads as wit and the audience just grabs on for the ride. "Rubies" as roller coaster! My husband, having spotted NYCB artistic director Peter Martins in the audience, said, "I bet he's poppin' a cold sweat."

I did not care for Svetlana Zakharova, who had the opening night "Diamonds." She is all extremes, with trick limbs that make one think of Sylvie Guillem, and a gluey plasticity that robs her dancing of spontaneity, accent. It doesn't help that she misses the mood swings in the music. Sofia Gumerova gave a persuasive reading on Saturday night, skating high on the icy surface of "Diamonds," a City Ballet display of swoop and scale. But it was Daria Pavlenko, Friday night, who was the sensation.

Pavlenko is a beauty, with a face of Art Deco exoticism as if drawn by Erté. Though offstage she's small as a mosquito, onstage she reads tall and has an endless line that could have come as well from Erté's pen. But she doesn't overplay that line. Pavlenko is one disciplined dancer, and she brings her own hushed momentum to the stage. Her "Diamonds" was all about hearing—the horns in the distance, the woodwinds rising, her own beating heart. She gave us wind shears of emotion in steps wholly performed. Her fourth positions on pointe, huge and deeply crossed, were displays of majestic chiaroscuro. Her *sous-sus*, tight as a top, were star bright and absolutely still ("at the still point, there the dance is"). And her arabesque—a gleam in the galaxy. In everything Pavlenko did she was thrilling. But this, after all, is what a ballerina must be.

So what would Mr. B think of how seriously the Kirov takes certain formalities, the polish this brings to the ballet? That I can't guess. But the pas de trois in "Emeralds," which the Kirov danced like three young purebreds trained and reined together, it was delight every time, an emperor's entertainment. And the four boys in "Rubies"—their uniformity of accent! They held formation like four wheels on a roadster, and revved up together like Hell's Angels at a stop sign. I love the way they drove through. And the corps and courtiers in "Diamonds." Under a blast of white light, and in white satin and tulle, the finale becomes a white act of its own, a union between two companies, a cosmic connection—"what might have been and what has been." This court climax is an evocation of the St. Petersburg of Balanchine's dreams, the snowbound palaces and Tolstoyan balls. To see it danced here by the company of those dreams, and with such inborn symmetry and ascendance, was like standing in the wings with Balanchine and seeing what he once saw.

It would be easy to use Kirov dancing as a stick with which to hit New York ballet companies. The Kirov arrived at the end of an ABT spring season of tired repertory, undistinguished (because one-dimensional) dancing, and too many principal women pushed beyond their talent (or unable to give because so unguided). Over at NYCB, a company bred for stylistic coherence, I saw a *Vienna Waltzes* in which the dancers were having trouble waltzing, let alone waltzing as one. And even among the most gifted young women at City Ballet, the dancing has gotten too thin, too divorced from fantasy, coquetry, poetry, love. This is why the company can't successfully cast a ballet like *Mozartiana*, a reliquary of all Balanchine believed in, a last masterpiece choreographed for Suzanne Farrell. The above-mentioned properties are each implicit in this ballet, and it is blind ideology to think they're not. It is also well to remember that Farrell, while rather bare branches up top, had a whorling volume from the belly down, a ripple effect that filled the eye and flooded the stage.

What we're seeing now is an odd reverse. Almost twenty years after Balanchine's death in 1983, we can't ride his coattails with such superiority. Our companies are in the same boat as the Kirov—no living choreographer of genius—but unlike the Kirov, our directors can't seem to bring up new ballerinas, at least not in such blissful batches. And where the Kirov has all of Balanchine to explore, so many NYCB dancers look all stretched out in him, with no place to go. And yet we continue to condescend, with the bean counters pointing out which step the Russians did wrong, which pose was not held long enough—missing the forest for the twig—and the village explainers trotting out Cold War clichés for a new generation, nonsense like: Russians go from pose to pose; or, Russians do squatty preparations for pirouettes (not true anymore, but everyone does a noticeable prep when the phrasing requires it, even Balanchine dancers). And here's one: If the Russians of the Mariinsky watch us enough they'll learn how to dance. Actually, maybe it's time for us to watch them.

Nestled within those three *Jewels* was a Saturday matinee *Swan Lake*. I dread *Swan Lake* these days. You almost never see much company connection to the work any more, or imaginative thrill in the dancing. The search for relevance—with settings in different eras, or sexy new gender transpositions—is often little more than hip subversion or a marketing ploy (or both), a way to whip up interest for next year's subscription series. The staging presented by the Kirov, however, was standard Sergeyev, with no outlandish interpolations or outré sets. Just a Saturday matinee *Swan Lake*.

After the curtain came down on Act Two, I walked up the aisle for intermission and felt something strange: contentment. The pas de trois, which dancers usually treat as a career move, intense and flashy, was danced by Scherbakov, Sologub, and Ekaterina Osmolkina with such faultless plush and gracious phrasing that it really did feel like a toast to civilized pleasures. And Veronika Part—it wasn't a show-stopping Odette, but a fascinating one. That heavy lightness of hers, so appropriately sinking into a dream in "Emeralds," was here a problem to be solved, a wreath of languor from which to break free. Part's bust, plummy feminine flesh in the manner of Ingres, seemed the stronghold of her mystery. She spoke with breast and back, plunging, twisting in her bodice—Odette as deep décolletage.

After Act Three, again a daze of wonder. The national dances, in which we look so forced, were riveting because the dancers know how to perform a czardas, a mazurka, how to toss their heads and wear their gloves and slide a foot on the floor as if slitting open a letter with it. In Russia it's their job to know these things. (The former Kirov dancer Vadim Strukov, an acclaimed character dancer, says of the mazurka, "It takes eight years in school to learn it. You work on it like a dog, and then you get to the theater and they still might not let you do it.") And Part, she ate space as Odile, charging the stage, legs reaching like a racehorse, and her arabesques unfurling with a swift mass that seemed to pull her back and away from her desire, a complex physics I've never seen before. Still dazzled, I ran into the *Ballet Review* critic Don Daniels, who spoke of Part's lower center of gravity, and how it offered a range of movement properties—centrifugal pleasures—we don't get from our lighter, more linear dancers. Yes. Pleasures of pull, not push, the tide inhaling under the waves. Here was a compleat *Swan Lake*, meticulously prepared from the corps up, every curve in alignment, the elements understood, a world created by the latitudes and longitudes of classical technique, and Odette bound in that net, its queen.

September 2002

Sellin' Out

Twyla Tharp has been choreographing dances for almost forty years, and by this time she should be a mature artist, yet she is not. If your subjects are aggression and apocalypse, how much can you mature? The filmmaker Stanley Kubrick, who made a career of cool doomed odysseys, antic and antisocial destructions, what did he end with? *Eyes Wide Shut*, a last film in which he saw and said nothing, despite the fact that it was based on a story by the Viennese writer Arthur Schnitzler, seer into souls. In a film about the subtleties of desire inside and outside of marriage, Kubrick came up empty. But then, when you do aggression-apocalypse you tend to get machismo-misogyny for free. Has Norman Mailer ever written a mature novel? Sam Shepard, a mature play? In Kubrick women are dolly-girls or just not there; in Mailer they're bimbos and bitches. This sounds a lot like Tharp. What begins as a dynamic fact of life—the might of masculine energy, its will to power—becomes the only high worth having, a groove on existential extremes. Why question the high? It's simpler, more aesthetically liberating not to.

Twyla Tharp has a new work on Broadway called *Movin' Out*, a show about Vietnam set to old songs by Billy Joel. The cast consists of three men who are teenage buddies, the two women who are their girlfriends, and a chorus, or rather, corps de ballet, that fills the other roles. Like Matthew Bourne's *Swan Lake*, the erotic update that stormed Broadway four years ago, there is no spoken language in *Movin' Out*. Billy Joel's rock ballads are organized to give us time and place, a musical panorama that spans the late sixties to the early eighties. It's up to Tharp to tell the story in dancing and to make

Landscape with Moving Figures

that dancing theater. What she comes up with is *Deuce Coupe* meets *The Deer Hunter*. Eddie and Brenda and Tony and Judy and James graduate from high school, the boys ship to Nam, the girls wait or wander, James dies, Judy cries, the boys return wrecks, everybody finds closure. All this in Tharp's signature style: phallocentric, hyperactive, hostile.

If you were to divide Tharp's art into periods, change would be loaded at the front. You'd have (1) Angry Young Woman—the severe and monotonal dances Tharp did with women very early on; (2) Androgyny—men are admitted into the company and in the process gender boundaries, all boundaries, blur and Tharp's slippery style is born; (3) Angry Young Man—in 1973, for the Joffrey Ballet, Tharp choreographs *Deuce Coupe* to Beach Boys music and discovers her inner teenage boy.

There was always an element of mockery to Tharp. Wearing a mop-top Beatles haircut, she built her dance style on a whole array of tuned-out teenage antagonisms, moves that looked like adolescent fidgets and sneers, shrugs and double takes. When Tharp danced solos, it was often as if she was wearing an invisible set of headphones, or was just ignoring the music, dancing to her own zoned-out drummer. She stuck wiggles and squiggles on steps—a kind of coloring outside the lines—and loved to suddenly spaz in double-time, a musical impertinence that signaled her impatience with the status quo. And she choreographed in a bumptious stream of consciousness—a little bit Abbott and Costello, a little late Joyce, a fine line between hyperarticulate and just plain hyper.

Within the context of classical dance, Tharp's tactics and antagonisms cut deeper. Audiences took them in good humor, the way one accepts snotty cracks from stand-up comics. Tharp was turned on by arrogant energy, performance in extremis, and when in 1976 at American Ballet Theatre she got to draft off Mikhail Baryshnikov in *Push Comes to Shove*, she never looked back. Balanchine's "ballet is woman" be damned. Tharp was one of the boys, and her dances revolved around guy after guy—Baryshnikov then Kevin O'Day then Julio Bocca then Angel Corella then John Selya. She worked boxing, aerobics, and break dancing into her ballets, and in *Men's Piece* (1992) summed it up in a cri de coeur: "Who wanted to be a girl, anyway?"

Tharp has always had big ambitions, though I'm not sure when she got the idea she could tell a story. Abstraction is her sandbox, the arena of her Charles Atlas kick fests. Her most self-consciously classical ballets (usually set to stern old masters, very contrapuntal), with their swimmy symmetries and stuck-there posture, sometimes look like sand castles when the tide's come in, shape dissolving right before your eyes. Tharp likes to fight the elements, fight the music, fight the world. She's always been better as an "action" choreographer, sliding, flinging, slapping, dripping, driving dancers across the stage solo, in twos, in groups. She gives in to lulls and lyric idylls only to raise the sword once more, a dynamic we see endlessly in her duets, Apache dances in which couples exhaust themselves in domestic battle, only to recharge and battle again. But a story? When Tharp did a narrative ballet for ABT called *Everlast*, the plot was puerile—something about a boxer and an ingenue—and the expense of the production nearly broke the company (when Tharp wants money she has a way of getting it).

The overture to *Movin' Out* is the song, "It's Still Rock and Roll to Me," which could be words from Tharp's mouth. And if we miss the reference to that first hit, *Deuce Coupe*, a dusty red convertible is wheeled onstage to remind us (it's totemic, like the obelisk in Kubrick's *2001: A Space Odyssey*). The characters announce themselves like dancers in *Hullabaloo*—Mouseketeers all grown up and doin' the Frug. As Eddie, John Selya in jeans greets us with a spate of delighted pelvic thrusts; Elizabeth Parkinson's Brenda shimmies onto the stage as if out of a go-go cage; Keith Roberts's Tony is Italian beef; Benjamin G. Bowman's James channels John Boy (natch, he dies); and Ashley Tuttle as Judy is his gumdrop of a girlfriend, pink and a little sticky. The band inhabits a high-tech catwalk above the action, blasting out Billy Joel oldies but goodies that are sung in a Joelesque voice by Michael Cavanaugh.

In the program, Tharp credits her son Jesse Huot "for having the idea for this show in the first place," and one can see that on paper it probably looked like a good idea, a return to her roots. She'd choreographed the movie *Hair* in 1978, she collaborated with David Byrne on *The Catherine Wheel* in 1981, and come on, Mom, look how well this retro stuff does on Broadway—*Grease*, *Mamma Mia*,

Hairspray—if anyone should be cashing in, you should. And why shouldn't Tharp marshal her forces and have a hit?

The problem is, when it comes to constructing characters she hasn't any forces to marshal. In one little dream ballet, Agnes de Mille could give us character on the couch, the vanities and fears, the catch of longing, the glint of a second, third, thought. Jerome Robbins could do it too, only glossier, snazzier. Tharp has never been able to do this. It's too small, too still, too close, too warm, too woman. It's just not her macho MO. And while those choreographers worked in other vernaculars, Tharp does not. One cannot imagine her dropping her tics and schticks to make dances for Tuptim. She has one vernacular: Tharp. Take it or leave it. So Eddie and Tony and James get a lot of whipping turns and judo leaps, and also that vaudeville-patter-camaraderie that Tharp trots out in the same cheapo way Woody Allen, when he needs a laugh or an answer, trots out clips of the Marx Brothers. As for Brenda and Judy, the beauty and the goody-good, they're so stock you could blow the dust off them. In almost forty years, Tharp still hasn't learned how to show us a female face.

If the characters are cardboard, then stagecraft could make the difference. All those decades in the theater should count for something. But in the few moments when a choreographic vision kicks in, *Movin' Out* doesn't look like Tharp at all, it looks like Paul Taylor, whose company Tharp danced in before she set out on her own. *Sunset*, *Company B*, one feels both of these Taylor masterpieces—evocations of war and what it does to love—sitting on Tharp's shoulders. In fact, the use of men in silhouette in a dance of mourning, or the way the corps is used in frieze patterns (very un-Tharp) to fill the stage and give battle action ballast, these moments look lifted. It isn't pretty, Tharp taking from Taylor this late in the day. Then again, Taylor would have chosen only five or six songs, would have concentrated in twenty-five minutes what Tharp has forced into and strung out for one hundred and twenty. He would not have betrayed songs by making them move in narrative directions they don't want to go or carry heavier emotional baggage then they can bear, as Tharp does with "She's Got a Way" and "Pressure." And he wouldn't have asked Ashley Tuttle to fake cry like a bad soap-opera actress. He would have given her dignity in loss. In a dance.

Movin' Out is as dated as an old yearbook, and as square, which is amazing from Tharp, the eternal tough. In the first section, with high school over and before the boys are drafted, it's *American Graffiti* does *American Bandstand*. In the war scenes, *Full Metal Jacket* morphs into *Miss Saigon*. When dead soldiers rise to do a ghost dance (a shameless gimmick), it's *The Night of the Living Dead* meets "Thriller." How faux is this show? When one of the songs ends with James blown away, bloody, twitching on the floor in a full-body death rattle, the audience applauds because it's the end of the song and because it's such virtuoso twitching. The crowd's hip to Tharp. *Movin' Out* is like MTV. You watch it with eyes wide shut.

December 2002

Bubble Boy

Mark Morris's arrival on the New York dance scene was spectacularly timed. George Balanchine died on April 30, 1983, leaving a company shaken, a following forlorn, and an art form facing a new era: classical dance post-Balanchine. Nine months later, on January 2, 1984, Mark Morris was born in the pages of *The New Yorker*, in a key-to-the-city review by Arlene Croce titled "Mark Morris Comes to Town." The timing was elegant, just the kind of fateful precision that served Balanchine during a long life of ups and downs, decisions and revisions. And the timing was comforting, not least because it was so Balanchinian. New York dance—stripped of its genius, its prize, its lyric lord—needed a reason to keep going. And here he was, a new genius: chewy, cherubic, with pre-Raphaelite ringlets and a dimple in his chin. Morris wasn't classical, he didn't make ballets. He was a modern dancer who drew from a variety of disciplines—folk dance, clog dance, high modern, postmodern, and, yes, classical (he performed with the Eliot Feld company for a time). And he was mightily musical in a showy way, using canon and counterpoint with amazing authority for one so young, an authority that made you think of Mr. B. Indeed, Morris forged the link himself in 1982. Without ever having seen Balanchine's *Liebeslieder Walzer*, Morris choreographed a dance to some of the same Brahms music and called it *New Love Song Waltzes*. Writing of the work in her 1984 review, Croce called it "the piece that most of Morris's admirers love best, and the one that stunned me with its precocity." Peter Martins, once precocious too, had ascended into Balanchine's position at the top of New York City Ballet, but it was Mark Morris, a modern dancer, who was the darling of the dance press, its foundling prince. In his 1984 solo *O Rangasayee*, he even wore a diaper.

O precocity. Morris was fresh in both senses of the word. Certainly no classical choreographer would have made an attempt on Balanchine's Brahms, a piece of music Balanchine came to in 1960, when he was fifty-six and in one of his glorious full-moon phases. His *Liebeslieder Walzer* is a drawing-room romance fit into a fine gold pocket watch, its four couples in white gloves circling their interior dramas—the erotic nature of each relationship—in 3/4 time. Morris's Brahms is more like summer camp after lights out. It isn't coupled, isn't straight or gay, but instead has a hum of the polymorphous perverse, as if any coupling is possible in the bushes by the lapping of the lake. Side by side, the two Brahms dances embody very different orientations. Balanchine explores individuals, giving us eight close-ups, eight characters waltzing around their private truths. Morris creates a faceless *La Ronde*, a twilight tumescence. He cuts against the text of love with a subtext of lust, an articulation of Puck's "what fools these mortals be," only Morris, warmer, is saying, "what humans . . ." He might even be saying, "what children . . ." Morris dancers have always had the look of barefoot kids whose big bodies have developed before they quite know what to do with them (they're costumed like kids, too, in underwear or untucked jammies or skimpy shifts or baggy tops and bottoms).

Where Balanchine's musical refinement was answered with dancing of like refinement—a classical technique of purring power, cat-lick finish, and emotion sensitively pitched—Morris's musical refinement served dancing that was blunt, earthy, purposely unpedigreed: legs unstretched, feet floppy and slappy, the upper body not lifted but just plumped there, undancerly, like any office worker. This very deliberate, often coarse, mind-body contrast could work wonderfully well, as in the early *Gloria*, a dance to Vivaldi in which spiritual prostration and sexual frustration knot up ecstatically. It could also look camp, which was no problem because Morris was pretty campy himself, his humor sort of Looney Tunes (when he bats his eyes at the audience, Morris is as faux femme as Bugs Bunny in drag). And it could look like nothing at all, as in a dance called *Behemoth*, a big, heavy, empty

Merce Cunningham knockoff that just stands there with a leg dangling in the air.

In the beginning, Morris was often compared to Paul Taylor, partly because Taylor has always liked robust bodies on his dancers (except Taylor dancers look like adults, not overgrown kids), and partly because Morris, like Taylor, was making dances that focused on the group at the expense of the individual. But there's a big distinction between the two. Taylor approaches populations, genres, as an anthropologist or scientist might, with a keen eye for their prevailing rules and postures, pacings and clichés, their ingrown way of dealing with sex and dissent, whether it be a colony of insects (*Counterswarm*) or a religious congregation (*The Word*). Taylor is tough, and he sees groups for what they are, not co-ops but tribes. Over and over he gives us the sacrificial lamb/maiden in his work: the crushing of the one for the good—the tradition—of the many. Mark Morris is into softer science. He's not an anthropologist, he's a sociologist, or, perhaps, a social worker. In the 1990s he did a dance called *The Office*, complete with a clipboard authoritarian: one by one the dancers were removed. In Morris's work, evil tends to come from without, not grow within, and so the group is an all-embracing place, a comfy commune, a pillow. This view hearkens back to Morris's early years with the Koleda Folk Ensemble.

"All the forms of happiness that he found in Koleda—artistic, social, emotional, physical—reinforced the communal vision," writes Joan Acocella in her 1993 biography, *Mark Morris*. "Utopianism is a constant theme of Morris's work, and that utopianism comes from Koleda." Morris's utopia is a charmed circle of equality and diversity, all body types and colors, no hierarchy of beauty, no stereotyping of gender. Basically, it's nurture versus nature, not the world as it is, but as it should be, an improvement upon it. This is not a metaphysics, it's a form of politics. And it is unique to the Mark Morris Dance Group.

It's important to remember that when Morris's company arrived in New York, something else had come to town, an epidemic called AIDS. People were terrified, nervous, depressed. As the eighties pulled on, the sadness in the dance community over Balanchine's death was joined to a greater, darker, deeper bereavement, the devastation of so many young lives lost, mostly men, many artists, dancers and choreographers among them. Openly gay from the start, with a musical gift that seemed Balanchinian, and a fondness for baroque music—the voice of the cathedral—Mark Morris was like a flame on the altar, a savior, a future, and it was during these years that he became a cult. Editors and critics fanned the flame, covering anything and everything he did. I fanned too. In fact, it was a curious phenomenon in which many dance writers let slip their critical distance so they might be just that: fans. There was safety in numbers, and the elation in the theater on those big BAM nights felt almost manic; those who did not join in were killjoys. "Lead us," sang the wavelength on the aisle. It was a huge and unfair burden to place on one artist.

Soon "us" was the Mark Morris audience, a clan that watches in high appreciation, brooks no criticism, and really gets the Bloomsbury–Barthes–*No Exit–Romper Room* wit, or rather, wink. Susan Sontag is its godmother; Sharon Delano its consigliere; *Threepenny Review*, the family paper; Isaac Mizrahi, its burbling bon vivant. It's an audience politically in tune with the whole utopia ethic, pleased with itself for being so in tune, ready to be pleased still more by whatever should happen onstage, surprisingly anti-analytical for a New York audience (despite Sontag, or maybe because of her), and always ready to laugh—I mean at anything. For some reason Twyla Tharp can fidget 'til she's blue in the face and no one finds it particularly funny. But if Mark Morris flips his hand spastically, as he did at predictable intervals in the recent dance *Foursome*, the audience guffaws. Every time. You can feel them ready and waiting, gathering for the next guffaw. In "The Latest Rage," a dead-on deconstruction of Morris's audience that ran in *Ballet Review*, Summer 2001, Michael Porter notes the "distinctive air of aggressive-passivity" and the "too facile embrace." Take that spastic hand flip. One sees that it doesn't relate to the music, doesn't correspond to a musical spasm. So it must be funny, because if it isn't funny then it's just . . . meaningless? A whim? Well, that's funny too: the Absurd. This audience invests heavily in these dances. As Porter reports in *Ballet Review*: "In the new illustrated monograph *Mark Morris's L'Allegro, Il Penseroso ed il Moderato: A Celebration*, the commentators on this particular work do not restrain their honorific comparisons. Among the artwork and artists invoked are Persian carpets, Beethoven's Fifth, *Ulysses*, Keats, Dante, Attic sculpture, Botticelli, Wagner's Ring Cycle, *The Four Temperaments*, Pasternak, Pushkin, *The Sleeping Beauty*, and Shakespeare's *A Midsummer Night's Dream*. Here empathy turns riot." In sixty-three years of dance-making Balanchine never knew such empathy.

So it's nineteen years since Mark Morris "came to town," nineteen years of prolific dance-making, partnership with Baryshnikov in the White Oak Dance Project, work with ballet and opera companies, and the building of his own school in Brooklyn. Mark Morris is now a brand and a business. But what about the dances?

I became disenchanted with Mark Morris in the 1990s. I tired of a gender neutrality that left women with the short end of the stick, mainly because the dances showed so little interest in *la femme* (these girls are kind of like Anybodys in *West Side Story*, heartfelt tomboys). And Morris's gift for metaphor began to seem played out, or perhaps abandoned, as if he was no longer interested in his most fundamental poetic device. Metaphor, after all, is artifice. It was increasingly clear that Morris's early work was his best work, and it never got better than *Dido and Aeneas*. Fascinating too, because *Dido* is the one big piece in which he plundered his hippie-dip utopia—in this case, Dido's kingdom—and did it with the joie de vivre of Don Giovanni adding another dumb broad to his list. It was a work in which Morris's dancers looked like adults—ironic, considering Purcell wrote the opera for a girls' school performance—and in which Morris's sensitivity to baroque music, his folk shapes and sturdy spatial constructions, not to mention his full-bodied aptitude for drag, all these talents dovetailed neatly to make an airtight expression: a work, a world, that contained its own seas and bed chambers and wind-snapped sails and Fates. It was a Greek myth built in one of Bruegel's beer bottles. Even Morris's use of mime, so often kindergarten simple, took flight as if against burnt-brown skies.

Dido and Aeneas premiered in 1989, four months after *L'Allegro, Il Penseroso ed il Moderato*, the dance Morris fans acclaim as his masterpiece. I suppose it comes down to cups of tea. To me, *L'Allegro* is another Morris dance that looks like it was made at summer camp. (Made at Jacob's Pillow would be better.) It has good things in it—some tight little pantomime sequences, very filigree—but so much of the rest is flat and runny pastel, like over-diluted watercolors being tilted on a board. Coy (I can't forget the circle of boys smacking each other's fannies), its garlanded gambols and euphoric running in rows become oppressively repetitive. If this is utopia, forget it. Maybe even Morris was sick of the softness; *Dido* seems to be made with wood beams and whalebone. Still, I agree that there's more invention in *L'Allegro* than in anything Morris is making today.

Most of what I've seen of Morris's choreography in recent years has been work outside his company. It isn't cheering. His stagings for opera often lack coherence. And his dances for ballet companies have been openly contemptuous of classical ambitions. Are ballet directors so hard up for choreographers, or just totally clueless? In *A Garden*, premiered by the San Francisco Ballet in 2001, Morris holds the dancers to the ground as if pinning down the corners of a tent. He allows them insipid leitmotivs that have no metaphorical spin or even juice and instead just leave you scratching your head. That spindly tendu with arms hovering waist level, stiff like a Barbie doll—why do we keep getting that pose? He shaves away hierarchy as if it were a wart. It's not only painful to see a willow like Muriel Maffre attempting to blend with the daisies in the corps, it's perverse. *Sandpaper Ballet*, worse still. Let's sand down the dancers, sand down distinctions. Everyone's dressed in green unitards, the grade-school green of modeling clay, and in drill formations they prance and wag rump en masse to the kitsch music of Leroy Anderson—Gumby does the Conga—all the while smiling like dopes.

Morris's *Gong*, premiered at ABT in 2001, is utterly confounding, a piece of chinoiserie for the corner cabinet, a better showcase for Mizrahi's costumes—tutus stiff as ceramics and tights with gold Hindu cuffs—than for dancers. They come out in rows and rows, Morris's favorite spatial strategy these days, and take turns hitting the same pose, one of those acutely mute positions Morris now specializes in, and that's the ballet. The only real dancing is in Michael

Landscape with Moving Figures

Chybowski's lighting—séance-like glimmers, the feel of things stealing in the night. In a way, Morris's performance on the PBS documentary *Born to Be Wild: The Leading Men of American Ballet Theatre* says it all. He clowns around. He doesn't act like a serious choreographer but like a kid, and he doesn't choreograph like a serious choreographer either. The piece he made for these four premier danseurs was bitsy busywork that said nothing about any of them, and didn't say much about Robert Schumann's music. It turns out that this little dance became "choreographic material" for the final movement of a larger dance, *V*, which makes you wonder if it ever had anything to do with ABT's men—and how deeply, for that matter, it has to do with *V*. Mark Morris, beloved for his endless invention, plopping a *pièce d'occasion* for ABT into a company work for his own dancers. How very communal.

I caught up with *V*—premiered in 2001 and pinned with critical corsages—at BAM last March. It was the last dance on a program that left me, one dance after another, acutely mute. Where to begin? With the audience I guess, that creepy tone of self-congratulation. Hey everybody, group hug.

The first dance, *Resurrection*, got reviews invoking film noir, murder mysteries, and Balanchine's Broadway ballet *Slaughter on Tenth Avenue* (both dances use the same music by Richard Rodgers). There is a couple, a backdrop with stars, and hands miming gunshots. But you have to imagine a noir wash over a sixties slumber party that's set, say, in a game-show studio. The dancers wear black-and-white pajamas in op art patterns (harlequins, squares, stripes), knowing toothpaste smiles are plastered on their faces, and then they're on the floor doing clumsy Busby Berkeley. A love story with no love, a murder with no death, it's a dream ballet with no dream, a Mark Morris so-what send-up.

Something Lies Beyond the Scene. If you would like to play skittles with Edith Sitwell, this one's for you. The music is William Walton's *Façade: An Entertainment with Poems by Edith Sitwell* (Sir Frederick Ashton choreographed the orchestral suite in 1931), and in this dance arch meets antic. See the boys and girls rushing about in T-shirts that sport cutesy symbols: duck, fish, suitcase, ear, cross, bird, boot. Sitwell's verse (read by Morris and friends in the pit), grotesque and tongue-twisty but every now and then sliding for seconds into grace, is mostly pretentious and unpleasurable, and so is the dance that goes with it. It's like an obscure semiotic scavenger hunt—the T-shirts, the Sitwell, the chesty air of understanding among the dancers—but what that semiotic something might be "lies beyond the scene."

Foursome. Four guys; Erik Satie; Judson Churchy; that spastic hand twitch. At this point I started wondering what people fifty years from now would make of these dances, the peculiar blend of humble pie and highfalutin. Will they see the affectless tone, arbitrary gestures, emotional void as wit?

V is set to Robert Schumann's Quintet in E flat for piano and strings, op. 44, a rather narrow and repetitive score. Morris answers that score with his watercolor formations and loose lines, though he can still be good with canon. *V* is in the vein of *Gloria* and *L'Allegro*, but it doesn't have a vocal text to swing on, and no gestures that catch and grow. The slow movement has dancers crawling across the stage like creatures pulling heavy loads—man as beast of burden—and it's another rough opposition. Yet Morris has done this so many times before. The dance goes on, the vision thins, running out long before the music is over. How weak Morris has become. Way back when, his work was defined by what it was: musically communicative, metaphorically alive. Now it feels like the sum of what it isn't, all those house rules against aesthetic conventions, cultural expectations, dance "lies" (his word) Morris won't tell. Funny how omissions have a way of growing into lies (never truths). So much effort to empty out, yet nothing much put back in. Morris could do a dance called *O*.

Two weeks before Morris's engagement at BAM, Paul Taylor's company performed at City Center. I won't go into the volcanic brilliance of *Last Look*, a dance from 1985 about humanity's last minutes on earth, a Spielbergian sky-ride through the final inferno, Taylor's dancers proving you don't need digital technology to show rolling backdrafts and gleaming meltdowns when you have a technique of such sandblast power and polish, and Michael Trusnovec the last man to see his face in a mirror, devolving before our eyes, Narcissus in Hell, a performance that was an assault on Patrick

Corbin's alpha stature within the company, and the dance a smoldering assault on euphemisms like "collateral damage," not because Taylor made it that way but because that's what art does, it speaks without being spoken to.

I won't go into Taylor's premiere *Dream Girls*, set to barbershop quartet songs, a piece so un-PC in so many directions it seems to be tweaking earnest downtown dance, but spinning out with such complete mastery of turn-of-the-century vernacular—low vaudeville and high burlesque—it's bliss.

I only want to mention one moment in Taylor's other premiere, a dance that could have been called "V" for the way it begins in V formation and continually returns to that V—but is titled *Promethean Fire*—a dance that looks like the inside of Radio City Music Hall, curve-on-curve Art Deco reverberation, and the outside of the Chrysler Building, aspiration piercing the sky; the dancers one minute heavy as chunks of marble, the next blizzarding into a fugue state (the music is Bach's Toccata and Fugue in D Minor); and Taylor playing fast and loose with heavy and light, sculpted and blurred, order and chaos, life and death and life. Patrick Corbin and Lisa Viola are the lead couple and in the middle of the dance they perform a leap and catch unlike any I've ever seen. It's the size, the scale, of something pair skaters do, the man tossing the woman up into the air and she spinning and landing a good ten feet away on one blade, only here it is done in reverse. Viola runs toward Corbin, throws herself into a jeté *en tournant* of such flying height that the entire audience lifts with her, and then lands low in Corbin's arms in a sweeping stag position, her leg neatly folded. The exhilaration of it; the arc and turn in the air; the swaying kiss of the catch; the bravery of them both; the audience's answering gasp of pleasure; and the dance completed in a flash, a flight, its themes of reach, fear, and faith caught up, written on air as only dance can do—there was more generosity, more lived life, in that double dare than in all four of those Mark Morris dances. And there was happiness in the theater.

Happiness—artistic, social, emotional, physical—is palpably absent from Morris's recent work. Sadness is missing too. In truth, there's no real emotion. Does Morris derive pleasure making these dances? One doesn't see it. Add up all the arch absurdities, patty-cake postures, formalities dumbed-down, genres camped-up, nonsense pretending to insight, Pepsodent grins patronizing the music, and you have a choreographic realm that is completely artificial, a hybrid of the very artifice Morris originally sought to avoid. Only a self-congratulatory audience could enjoy this stuff, as it's the only audience that won't see what isn't there. Those who all these years have supported Morris with unconditional love—extravagant praise for middling effort, qualified praise for bad work—have hurt him. The boy's in a bubble. It's time for Mark Morris to bounce out of his sterile utopia and get some damned life back into his dances.

June 2003

Stromanizing

> *It takes hours daily of blind instinctive moving and fumbling to find the revealing gesture, and the process goes on for weeks before I am ready to start composing. . . . This is the kernel, the nucleus of the dance. All the design develops from this.*
>
> —Agnes de Mille, *Dance to the Piper*

To be a dancer in America in the thirties and forties—the decades when Martha Graham was moving earth with her flexed foot, Eugene Loring was playing Cowboys and Indians to Copland, Antony Tudor was pulling G-force expressionism from a classicism in stays, Jerome Robbins was coining character with a jukebox genius for vernacular, and George Balanchine was taking dictation from God (lightning speed, cat-paw quiet) and a footnote from Fred Astaire (that swingy, selfless style)—to dance was a vocation. No one has written better about the calling than Agnes de Mille, herself a groundbreaking choreographer in those landmark years. De Mille's books are gems of eyewitness reporting and insight, and especially radiant are the discussions she had with Graham, a best friend and very much the big sister. Their conversations were always about the search, the struggle, the "don't compromise," the divine, even if it was sometimes what Graham called "divine dissatisfaction, a blessed unrest that keeps us marching." Onward, Choreographic Soldiers.

"Quickening" was another Graham word, as in "a vitality, a lifeforce, an energy, a quickening." It too has a religious connotation, the moment, according to Aquinas, when a soul is divinely infused.

Remembering the breakthrough influence that Igor Stravinsky's *Apollon Musagète* had on him, Balanchine, in the 1940s, wrote, "I began to see how I could clarify, by limiting, by reducing what seemed to be multiple possibilities to the one which is inevitable." Call it what you will—"the revealing gesture" or "the one which is inevitable"—all the design develops from this. When Antony Tudor was making his 1942 masterpiece *Pillar of Fire*, "Hagar's gestures," de Mille reports, "were chosen with prayer and fasting." Trial by fire, gesture forged in fire, Promethean fire, art. Hagar's very first movement—which is the ballet's as well—opens her to the audience like nasty gossip. She is sitting alone on the front steps of a house and slowly her right hand, flat and tense as a blade, lifts from her lap toward her temple in a slow-motion scythelike arc and smooths her already smooth hair. She is wound tight, marking time, sick with its passing, nearly hopeless, and this slow seminal motion, the climbing flat of her hand, will grow into larger moves, will inflame in a series of bodily arcs and lunges, reaches and retreats, a tug of war between abandon and regret. And it all begins in the flat of the hand.

And then there's de Mille. One of the things I love about her work, especially her work on Broadway, is the way she found a wholehearted, almost reverential yet stylized in-between: a plastique that took a slightly off, but simple, move or pose or gesture and graced it—poeticized it—with the pulled-up, still-point energy of classical dance. No wonder she was such a perfect fit with Rodgers and Hammerstein; they, too, worked reverence, songs like steeples, into their musicals. De Mille was a great synthesizer. She learned from Graham and Tudor, worshiped their achievements, and partook—too much some say, though I don't—of what they created. De Mille's work has a weighted lightness, a low plumb that's not as heavy, pitching, as Graham's, and a plastique as taut as Tudor's, but shadowless, as if the sun is always high above. She's like milkweed; the pods are rough, brown, but the stem runs with whiteness and the seeds fly. Look at *Oklahoma!*, *Carousel*, *Brigadoon*—not just at the dream ballets—and you're blown away. Movement unfurls in fluttering bolts, and then it's cut for an ecstatic moment, a pose frozen like an action shot in a forties fashion magazine.

Landscape with Moving Figures

Example: Laurey's leap onto Curly's shoulder, like a doe on a cloud. You just gaze at how wonderful it is.

Is such stylization dated today? Three years ago at City Center, American Ballet Theatre's best effort was de Mille's *Rodeo*. Like a barn raising, sprung with air, the ballet just stands up before you. And because the characters are so true, their gestures like strikes of a silver hammer, the story tells itself through rhythm, grouping, and folk dance forms—no words necessary. It didn't hurt that in Joaquin De Luz, now a soloist at New York City Ballet, the company had an irresistible Champion Roper.

Last October at City Center, ABT revived Tudor's *Pillar of Fire*, a more difficult ballet all around, with Julie Kent, Gillian Murphy, and Amanda McKerrow having their first attempts at Hagar. Even if Kent hadn't been almost five months pregnant, she would have been miscast. Her Hagar was a spinster Juliet, stiff and prettified. Murphy danced with more muscle, but in a cowering way, as if Hagar were a victim, the subject of abuse. She's not. She's a soul on fire, a battlefield in her breast, desperate for love but in a moment of defeat willing to take just sex. Who hasn't been so torn? McKerrow's performance was smarter, more linear and coherent, but not deep or big enough, not enough in her eyes. *Pillar of Fire* is not just a story of small-town, ingrown judgment and sublimation, it is also about the making of an artist (it made Nora Kaye, the first Hagar). You must lose yourself to transcend yourself. The music, after all, is Schoenberg's *Verklärte Nacht* ("Transfigured Night"). *Pillar of Fire* is transfigured storytelling, even without a Hagar that burns bright. The shorthand is sharp, the narrative flow sure, cursive, one minute telescoped close in, the next swept off in the distance; we seem to move through a real town in real time, then suddenly the ballet is out of body, an erotic dream, innocence and experience dancing together, as if the town itself were dreaming of what happens at its edges in the dark. Oh for such storytelling today. It wasn't until I saw Susan Stroman's new work for New York City Ballet that I realized how much I miss the revealing gesture, the stylized soul quickening onstage.

Stroman's dance is the first of four works commissioned as part of NYCB's centennial celebration—the hundredth anniversary of

George Balanchine's birth in 1904. It's been eleven years since the last big celebration: in 1993, NYCB honored the tenth anniversary of Balanchine's death by performing, in chronological order, seventy-three of his 425 ballets. If that undertaking was sublime in scope, this one is on the skimpy side. I don't mind that. Balanchine, who liked to build festivals around composers (Stravinsky, Ravel, Tchaikovsky), probably would have waved away his 100th with a *Who Cares?* flourish—a vodka toast and on to 101. But what would he think if he got this for a present: a full-length ballet by a Broadway choreographer?

Not a *pièce d'occasion*. Not a thirty-minute movement sonnet, a pure dance project that the deep-pocket producers on 42nd Street would never get. No, Martins has given Stroman the whole stage for an entire program. Not even Jerome Robbins, the most brilliant Broadway choreographer of the last sixty years, and a resident choreographer at NYCB for many of those years, got the whole enchilada at the State Theater. Balanchine worked at full-length, but infrequently: *The Nutcracker*, *A Midsummer Night's Dream*, *Don Quixote*, *Jewels*, *Coppélia*. Peter Martins has added to that: his attractive if rather cramped *Sleeping Beauty* of 1991, his homely and stylistically inappropriate *Swan Lake* of 1999 (if you have Mr. B's take on the classic, you don't need Mr. M's). And now there's this, an outside effort called *Double Feature*, the title a reference to the silent movie format of Stroman's show. I can't bring myself to call it a ballet.

The rationale behind this commission, its connection to the centennial, is a glib byte. Peter Martins in *Playbill*: "In the thirties Balanchine was 'Mr. Broadway,' as was Jerome Robbins later on. Today, Susan is definitely 'Ms. Broadway,' so it seemed perfect to have her here this year to honor Mr. B's legacy as a Broadway pioneer." Never mind that the presence in rep of Balanchine's *Slaughter on Tenth Avenue*, his ballet from the 1936 musical *On Your Toes*, is enough for many of us (we all love *Slaughter*, we do, it's lots of fun, but I think I'll skip out on it tonight). Never mind that you can get your Broadway Balanchine in better places, like *The Four Temperaments* (those slow-motion kicklines), *Western Symphony*, *Stars and Stripes*, *Who Cares?*, the third part of *Union Jack* (there's a lot of Shubert Alley in those third-movement curtain closers), not

133

to mention "Rubies," a whole Broadway show in tiaras and red satin. Susan Stroman is currently the most award-winning choreographer on Broadway—five Tonys for starters—and that makes her a gold-plated prize in these days of risk-averse arts marketing. A couple questions, though. Is Martins simply ignoring the fact that Stroman is also the most overrated choreographer on Broadway? Or is he innocent of all that?

The great claim for Stroman is that she's a storyteller who tells the story "in dance." What I've seen of her work proves the opposite. Take away the sets, the spoken words, the projected titles, the heavy-handed visual and musical cues—take away the Broadway show around the dances—and there isn't much to differentiate her choreography in *Contact* from her choreography in *The Music Man* from her choreography in *Oklahoma!* from her choreography in *Double Feature*. Stroman travels light. She goes from project to project with two little bags: one holds her scant vocabulary of steps, the other her small number of tricks. You can get them all in *Contact*, the strange musical Stroman developed with Lincoln Center Theater, a show that wowed dum-dum theater critics and left dance critics cold. It has three acts/scenarios (perhaps they're supposed to be dream ballets), but the one where you see Stroman's vocabulary go all the way from A to B is the middle number, "Did You Move?"

Described as "fantasies of a downtrodden housewife in 1950s Queens," it begins with a couple sitting down for dinner in an Italian restaurant. The husband is a brute and the wife is a ditz, but a lonely ditz, browbeaten. Increasingly furious because he can't get a roll, the husband leaves the table from time to time to get more food or to look for a roll, admonishing his wife, "Don't talk, don't smile, don't fuckin' move." Every time he leaves the stage, his wife dances around the room—a fantasy, of course—trying to make contact (the title!) with other people. Is this description getting tedious?

Stroman's little bag of steps includes the following: a popped-up *développé à la seconde* (a high kick to the side), various jetés, skips, chassés (a kind of sliding gallop), pas de chat, pas de bourrée, and a textbook arabesque. These steps are linked together in combinations you might find in any adult beginner class at any ballet school in the country. They're over-emphatic, herky-jerky, the teacher keeping things big and bouncy for students not yet ready for nuance, the refinements begun at the intermediate level: feeling the psychological difference between *en dedans* and *en dehors* (inward and outward, darkness and light), finding the subtle shading of *épaulement* (that cameo intimacy of bust and head), climbing into the high altitudes of adagio—lift, hold, breathe, reach—those invisible mountain passes touched with eternity and pain. But getting back to *Contact*, why ballet? A housewife in 1950s Queens would be wearing a girdle, her deportment in the real-life moments would have a bit of ballroom formality, stillness. Shouldn't her dream dancing have something of that fifties formality? Gene Kelly romancing Leslie Caron? The silk of Cyd Charisse? Why is she hearing frantic classical music and not Rosemary Clooney, Frank Sinatra, Nat King Cole, those fireside classics? When she's felt up by a waiter under the table, it's a disconnect: Is this the wife's fantasy of romance or Stroman's idea of humor? "Did You Move?" is a coarse and sophomoric piece of theater, and it's bad dance.

The third act of *Contact*—the "Girl in Yellow" section—is also coarse, and almost endless, but choreographically it's an improvement. Stroman is held within the grooves of swing dancing, line dancing. This helps, because it forces upon her the act, in Balanchine's words, of "limiting . . . reducing what seemed to be multiple possibilities." Well it's something. Still, the two main characters, potential lovers, are the broadest of stereotypes, he the isolated workaholic, she the cool beauty. They never quicken into something we can care about because they haven't one revealing gesture between them.

Here's an experiment you can do at home. Rent both the 1955 film of *Oklahoma!* (Shirley Jones and Gordon MacRae; choreography by de Mille) and the 1999 revival, just released (Josefina Gabrielle and Hugh Jackman; choreography by Stroman). About fifteen minutes in you'll find the ensemble number "Everything's Up to Date in Kansas City." Look at the differences. De Mille has blond Gene Nelson as Will Parker, the character just back from winning a rodeo in K.C. She's got him in cowboy boots, tight pants, and a black hat—already he's stylized, heightened like a flamenco dancer, slim as a spike. Yet how does the number begin? With Nelson in a catcher's

Landscape with Moving Figures

squat, off to the side by a wood crate. So it begins quietly, Nelson planted low, then rising on stovepipe legs, walkin' that cowboy walk, singin' about what he's seen (Gas buggies! Burleycue!), then back down into that sexy squat, pants taut across his thighs, as if the dance is warming up and taking its time. You feel that—acres of time and everyone quiet in the sun, watching Will. He does a two-step in a circle, exaggerating it, but his second pass, a ragtime tap, that's more his style, a riding style from the hip down, quiet through the leg, giddyup in the heel. He keeps circling, his tapping clipped as grass, each pass more complicated, but always returning home to that crate on the side. Even when the other cowboys join in and de Mille brings the dance to a boil, double-time and breakaways—two girls, an old woman, and all these rough men—it's friendly, orderly, always within the hub, the homemade decorum and dishtowel snap of that communal circle. Will Parker, our hayseed Apollo with the beautiful thighs, is the kernel of the dance.

Stroman, in her version, takes Will Parker out of boots and puts him in brown flats so long they almost look like clown shoes. She has him demonstrating bawdy dance-hall moves, among them her favorite funny step, the recurring Stroman Squat: second-position plié on tiptoe, done fast and goosey (it's totally wrong for a cowboy, even a chorus-boy cowboy). Stroman stages "Kansas City" as a loud, rowdy number, a free-for-all. There's no communal center, no developing design, no feeling of land or love for Will (this one's so charmless he's almost a clod), just one stunt after another—rope tricks, backflips, split jumps, wham bam thank you ma'am. Stroman doesn't grow a dance, she Stromanizes the stage, empties her bags of bombast on the music. When it's over you're flattened.

Double Feature is prefab theater, smooth on the surface, no foundation down below. It consists of two acts—a melodrama called "The Blue Necklace" and a comic romp called "Makin' Whoopee!"—which tell their stories through the conventions of silent movies, i.e., projected dialogue, lots of props, and the implied lyrics of the popular songs that make up both scores. Ballets aren't supposed to need so many words, or any words at all. The whole point is that they communicate what words cannot. But Stroman the storyteller needs words, and thus the inter-title projections are lengthy and continual. You spend as much time reading as watching, and this is a cheat. Why grow a dance from the flat of your hand when you can have thoughts thrown on a screen above your head? Adding to the conceptual confusion (for me, anyway), when the movie-theater scrim lifts on "The Blue Necklace" we see a kickline of chorus girls on pointe at Valentine's Variety Theatre. So it's a ballet that's a silent movie about a vaudeville dancer who becomes a movie star. "They're chorines," a friend said wonderingly, "but they're in tutus?" The whole dimensional question is wonky-making, and Stroman might have played with it (as Paul Taylor did in his film-noir treatment of *Le Sacre du printemps*), finding a focus by acknowledging the question. But she doesn't. As usual, she just empties her two bags—steps and schtick—in the little bit of stage in front of the sets. It's all foreground, but then again Stroman's work is all foreground.

"The Blue Necklace" is a weepy that turns into a Cinderella story. An aspiring actress (or is she a dancer?) leaves her illegitimate baby girl and a blue necklace on a church step, the child is adopted by a man whose wife is the archetypal wicked stepmother, the actress becomes a star and wants to find her daughter, who grows up, goes to an orphans' ball sponsored by the actress-mother, proves her DNA by dancing well, and blah-blah-blah happy ending. The score is Irving Berlin hits arranged by Glen Kelly, nicely done but way too long. Doug Besterman's orchestrations are accomplished, yet from the very first notes you hear a pushy, almost presumptuous tonal appropriation of Hershy Kay's medley of Gershwin for *Who Cares?* Riding coattails, nostalgia by numbers, whatever. It's too much and too easy. Robin Wagner's scenery is precise, the source of the show's sleek feel.

As for Stroman, her work with a classical vocabulary is not worthy of this stage. She keeps the dancers moving, keeps going and going, trying to coin a phrase, find a flow, a momentum, a meaning. I think that's why every solo and duet goes on too long, with louder repeats: she knows the steps aren't moving the story. At the orphans' ball, watching the belaboring of Berlin's "The Best Things Happen While You're Dancing," all I could think of was the 1954 film *White Christmas*. Rent it and see what Robert Alton, a real Broadway choreographer, did with Danny Kaye, Vera-Ellen, a dock

Landscape with Moving Figures

outside a dinner club, and that song. Talk about phrase and flow. Later on, Stroman does well with "Mandy," using it to introduce the matinee idol danced by Damian Woetzel. The dance is light, skipping, rhythmically acute, and it has personality, suggesting a man who skips through life and is quick to shine. It's a narrowing in that opens out.

Stroman makes a lot of references to older ballets, shows, choreographers. You could call her (and some do) Ms. Pastiche. Why hasn't she learned what goes into the crafting of these classics? Watching her Stromanize "Marian the Librarian" in the revival of *The Music Man*, I felt like yelling, "Grab a dictionary and look under S for *stylized*, *subconscious*, *subtext*, or *symbol*." In the famous essay quoted earlier, Balanchine writes that he came "to understand how gestures, like tones in music and shades in painting, have certain family relations. As groups they impose their own laws." In "The Blue Necklace," Stroman should have shown us the "family relation" between mother and daughter, not from the outside with subtitles and cues, but from the inside, kinetically, with something they share like a genetic code—the inevitable step, a revealing gesture.

One of Stroman's most dependable tricks *is* kinetic. It's not so much a one-two effect as a twofer, a split second in which two things happen at once. *Contact*: husband drops his plate on the table/wife whips a napkin off her head. *Oklahoma!*: trunk glides in out of nowhere/Will Parker lands on it just as it stops. These twofers are percussive punctuation, like exclamation marks, and good for making nothing happening seem like something happening; in short, good for Stromanizing. Sometimes, though, the exclamation speaks. In "The Blue Necklace," the adopted daughter dances around the living room she's supposed to be cleaning, and every time the mean mother bursts in the daughter falls to the floor pretending to scrub. It's a funny bit, explosive in the right way, and oddly touching because we begin to see character shown not told.

"Makin' Whoopee!," using the songs of Walter Donaldson, is based on *Seven Chances*, a Buster Keaton movie about a young man who will inherit millions if he can marry by seven that night. I can just hear Stroman selling it to Martins, something like, The chase scenes, all those girls in bridal gowns, it's the Wilis in *Giselle*. If only this piece

138

had been half as long as it is, a two-reeler, so that Stroman could have concentrated her slim resources on the slim story. Alexandra Ansanelli and Tom Gold are wonderfully cast, a little wedding-cake couple, and Gold especially has a triumph as the unblinking Buster Keaton, a yearning romantic trapped in the black cloud of his dark suit, his body always a beat behind his heart. But again, Stroman pads it out. The pas de deux in the park, where the Keaton character proposes to various females, are tiresome. The dances for Gold and his two business partners, a real Broadway trio, should be wittier, more inventive, with more of those twofers. They never quite click in. And why does Stroman have Gold, who's clearly worked hard to get the Keaton plastique, suddenly toodling around like Chaplin's Little Tramp? ("'Cause she always throws in the kitchen sink," said a theater queen I know.) The climactic chase is a coup de théâtre. The stage is clear and a mass of brides-to-be pound after Gold in long thick diagonals. It's always fun to watch people run, really run, onstage. Some of the brides are guys in drag, and when one of them falls down under a strobe effect it gets a huge laugh. A little dog, a Boston Terrier, gets an even bigger laugh. Leaving the theater I thought, Wouldn't it be great to have a Boston Terrier?

I've asked friends in the theater why Stroman is so dominant on Broadway when the work is so undistinguished. I always get the same answer: She's easy to work with, a team player, she doesn't storm the director with demands, she's nice. Suddenly the baseball hat makes sense—the black baseball hat, one of the boys, that is Stroman's signature accessory. In other words, she's not a Beelzebub like Robbins, purgatory on two legs (but his shows are shot with heat and light). She's not a pain in the ass like de Mille, famous for her tantrums, those biblical floods of tears (but the dances are icons of American history). And she's not a Graham, who broke rule after rule in her quest never to lie, the first rule broken, according to de Mille, "that of being a good egg—one of the gang."

Dance is not a gang or a team. It is a vocation. You must lose yourself to transcend yourself. Susan Stroman, Ms. Broadway, has five Tonys and counting. What she doesn't have is a moment of truth.

March 2004

Assoluta

Divas are a dime a dozen. Pop singers are divas, actresses are divas, models, anchor ladies, female CEOs, even women who snap at cabbies are divas. The term *diva* has its most revered usage at the opera, where it is enshrined in a spectral aria—"Casta diva"—sung by Norma, the title character in Vincenzo Bellini's masterpiece. Norma is a Druid priestess who, trapped between duty and desire, goes up in flames for love, a flashpoint you might say, for the kind of power that now dominates in America: dark power, chthonic power, the id simmering, "issues" spitting, entitlement and empowerment stirring in the brew. There is something of witchcraft about divas. Singers plant themselves onstage (think of Judy Garland's wrestler's stance) and pull up their arias through the ground, the gut, the ribcage, the throat. Incanting, decanting, they obsess about phlegm and sediment, fearing they will open their mouths and hear nothing, the cauldrons below gone cold (Kathleen Battle, a diva well named, threw fits if anyone looked at her lips). Temper is never plucked from blue sky.

Great female ballet dancers are not called divas, or even prima donnas, though they may act that way. They are ballerinas. Or prima ballerinas. Or prima ballerina assoluta—it doesn't go any higher. And yet these glorious titles have gone out of use. It is now only and simply ballerina.

Ballet dancers pull up too. It is part of the technique. The five positions of ballet—positions of the feet and the alignment of the body over them—are primary placements, architectural foundations. But they are not dug in, planted. In any position, weight must hover, angelically poised, above the balls of the feet. In this way the dancer is ready, like a dandelion puff in a breeze, to lift in any direction—light, effortless, a different kind of power. Classical ballet is not earth and fire, it is water and air, the dewpoint of a culture. Ballerinas are not bitches throbbing out molten wants and recriminations (though in postmodern ballets they're often asked to stomp and throb). They are cultivated like pearls or white peacocks or royal roses. They are trained on the luminous. National treasure and north star, the ballerina is informed by all the arts—music, painting, poetry, fashion, as well as *la danse*—with a little Euclidian geometry as underpinning. Moth wing and spider's web are her adornments, a toilette of tulle and tiara. As for the fairies, sylphs, Wilis, and sprites that are so often her subject, well, today we understand that these folklore apparitions are not so much tricks of the eye as they are events of energy, thermodynamic transmutations—flash, blur, ripple, wave—a healthy wood or meadow in a split-second bliss of iridescence, a shiver of pleasure escaping. This is what a ballerina must be, an event of pure unplanted energy, and why she is so rare.

Today, the term itself is slippery. The general public thinks any girl who makes a living in toe shoes is a ballerina. Subscribers, a bit smarter, assume that the top of the roster—principal dancers—are the ballerinas, though it is wrong to think they are simply corps girls grown up; the mark of the ballerina is often perceived way back in the academy, where one girl is already different, more, than her peers. Balletomanes like to play with the word, sometimes using it to describe an aura of romance or theatricality. "He's not strong," I once heard it said of the French dancer Alexandre Proia, who wore his hair like Liszt, "but he's a real ballerina." Then again, it's not unusual to hear a 'mane despair, deadly serious, of a major ballet company, *"But they have no ballerinas."* Which is not to say the company is without stars. You can be a star without being a ballerina (just look at American Ballet Theatre's Paloma Herrera), and today there are many ballet stars trouping the world's stages (just not many ballerinas).

The late David Daniel, a dance and music critic of easy erudition, had a particularly withering phrase for the classical dancing he was seeing at the end of the twentieth century. "But you know, dear," he would say, "it isn't dancing. It's what I call"—and here the poison pause—"*doing* ballet." That glib verb redolent of corporate lunches and busy-bee lists—to do. For David there was an unbridgeable difference between dancing and doing, between artistry and athletics, art and airs, a dancer answering the history encultured in her muscles and one who hears little, who gives a silhouette of a performance, a facsimile, all steps accounted for, a face full of agony or ecstasy pulled on cue. It was the difference, finally, between going to the theater and staying home. "Have-a-nice-day ballet" is what the critic Joel Lobenthal calls it—dancing that is shiny, smiley, skinny.

In the seventies there was a corps dancer at ABT named Fanchon Cordell. I never saw her perform with the company, but I met her at the ballet studio of Albertine Maxwell in Nashville, Tennessee, where she took daily class with the advanced students while on a two-week visit home. Her presence was electric. We all worked harder trying to pull up to her level, to learn from her, secretly hoping to hear an encouraging word from this young woman who was the real thing. I vividly recall an afternoon in the dressing room when we gathered around and she talked about ABT, specifically of Natalia Makarova and Gelsey Kirkland, each having joined the company in the early seventies. Makarova's awesome flow, Kirkland's heartbreaking ardor—the arrival of these two women, Cordell explained, was a huge jolt to the company's female dancers. Everyone, she said, worked harder. Makarova and Kirkland, each in her own way, showed how much more one could give.

What is that *more*? With Kirkland it was a commitment that came across the footlights, a mighty myopia in that babydoll face. Kirkland was trained at the School of American Ballet and came of age at the New York City Ballet. Rebellious since a child, she couldn't see her way to George Balanchine's rule, "Don't think, just dance." Not thinking was not in her nature. Kirkland joined ABT where her relentless thinking about her dancing, her seeking after its soul with coach after coach, her quest for meanings in a wordless form, all this desire gave charging grandeur to her dewy pointillist precision. Walk into the Jerome Robbins Dance Division at the Lincoln Center Library and somewhere in the room, on one of the video screens, a young dancer will be viewing the 1978 Kirkland-

Baryshnikov performance of *Theme and Variations*. Misha is wonderful in it, but he's not the reason they're watching. It is Kirkland, dancing in the crystal castle of her technique, meticulous, swift, a silvery joust, her French twist gleaming, her hummingbird heart full and pumping. You feel the moat of air around her, see the prismatic transcendence within, her energy so much higher, hotter, more pure than Misha's. "Gelsey always looked like she was beamed in from another planet," my husband remembers. "She was like a hologram." Exactly. She *was* from another planet, each performance a visitation, a fresh search for answers. Indeed, one of Kirkland's early answers was Makarova—inspiration and jolt. Kirkland admits she imitated Makarova's seamless line; she could not imitate her Vaganova Academy training, hence the need for teachers.

Makarova didn't lay her heart so plainly before the audience, perhaps because she'd grown up with the answers. At the Imperial School of the Mariinsky Theatre, questions of meaning ("Is Prince Siegfried reading Shakespeare or Lermontov?") were debated after class. And Makarova knew—because it's in the Kirov curriculum, hence culture, to know—every interlocking level of theater, from the right way to breathe, to how to rescue a step, to the dramatic verities of the great ballets, for instance, that the role of Giselle is not a series of set pieces but a single phrase that goes from sun to sun, a long arc of ever more out-of-body implosions (yes, the ballerina must dance a contradiction). Where Kirkland's Giselle was a psychosexual fever, all that anxiety and longing compressed, Makarova's was a kinetic surrender, an artist bringing a supreme simplicity into the darkened passage of Act Two. It was a performance built on ballon and on the catching momentums of a breathing *épaulement*, so soft it seemed to be all essence, the murmuring energy of Kirov generations: illumined, lunar, a rising fealty, then sinking into darkness, the woods, which is of course what happens in *Giselle*. At the ballet, imagination and energy are the same shape, the same property. When these women were onstage you never wondered, as one so often does today, why they were the standard—the ballerinas.

This spring season at the Metropolitan Opera House, ABT staged a new production of *Raymonda*, Marius Petipa's full-length ballet of 1898. It's a strange ballet, famous for its glorious score by Alexander Glazunov, and infamous for its story, the view being that it's thin (Balanchine called the story "nonsense"). In Act One, Raymonda celebrates her birthday; pines for her betrothed, Jean de Brienne, who is off fighting the Crusades; receives a tapestry portrait he has sent of himself; then takes a nap and dreams first of Jean and then of the Saracen chief, Abderakhman, who is wooing her in Jean's absence. In Act Two, Jean comes home and wins Raymonda back, defeating the Saracen in a duel. Act Three is the marriage celebration. *Raymonda* is a bit like *The Sleeping Beauty* (the dream scene works like *Beauty*'s vision scene; the male lead arrives late), only without the fairy-tale balance, the twin peaks of Lilac Fairy versus Carabosse. In fact, except for the duel, *Raymonda* seems to go from valley to valley, the score less a narrative with a feisty through-line than a collection of ballads, reveries, dreams, hummingly lovely. Ballet emerges from the quiet of a culture, and the ballerina from a quiet of her own creation; you could say *Raymonda* is about nothing less than this. It is a landscape of Raymonda's contentments, desires, and fears, her interior life in a tutu. The role has five solos and four codas, a number that looms, and all are laid bare, no plot twists or mad scenes from which to draw color or camouflage. She's alone with the character of her dancing.

It's amazing, in a bad way, how long a shortened full-length ballet can feel. As is the trend at both ABT and NYCB, this new *Raymonda* was parcelled around one intermission, making for long sits on each side. What story there once was is now so cut, futzed with, and abridged the ballet feels more like a *Raymonda* hit parade. But at least it's pretty. Zack Brown brings a touch of twilight to his Arthurian sets, veiled layerings in frost blue, lavender, persimmon— William Morris medieval—and it works against the concert-version flatness of the production, plumping it up. His costumes remind me of Adrian's wonderful work for Lerner and Loewe's *Camelot*—"confectioner's gothic" it was called. Disturbingly, Anna-Marie Holmes and Kevin McKenzie have done away with the symbolic tapestry that prompts Raymonda's dream. In this version, Jean de Brienne is no longer crusading during Act One; he's made it to Raymonda's birthday where he hangs around so long he doesn't seem special anymore. Meanwhile, Raymonda never has to long for him, or suffer she may have lost him, a fear that leaves her naked to the Saracen. Now she's just another dumb birthday girl. The whole emotional plumb is lost, the weight of the place Raymonda visits in her dream, in her heart. Gone too an epic sensibility, the land waiting for Jean's return. So much pointless alteration here, or perhaps preemptive, as if to protect ABT's principal women, and maybe its audience, from a role that's too artistically revealing.

Of the performances I saw, ABT's Raymondas were all over the map. Xiomara Reyes, a cloying dancer whose principal status baffles me, was without nuance or a glint of understanding. ABT's roster has always included one or another of these chirpy soubrettes, Junior Mints for the "Isn't she cute?" clucks in the audience. But to cast this type as Raymonda is ridiculous. And what does it say to the dancers below? That a Reyes Raymonda is good enough for management? That's the standard? Gillian Murphy, whom the company is promoting with great gusto, did better. She had pluck, more lightness than is her norm, and gave us . . . not a Raymonda, really, but a gutsy Aurora. Murphy is athletic, a natural turner, and the speed she brings to pirouettes, fouettés, *chaînés* is her specialty, so if it's speed you want, Murphy's your girl. But when she isn't pulled taut to the vertical, as dancers are during turns, problems blink at you: the blockiness in the body, knees that don't always straighten, the weak leg extension *en avant* ("forward"—in sheer physics the most difficult of all extensions, stumpy when badly done, a prophetic unfolding when strong). And then there's the stunning lack of melody in her dancing. Many think Murphy a virtuoso (it's the turns), but to my eye the dancing is clotted, technically thick. If the head cheerleader became a ballet dancer, she'd be Gillian Murphy.

Nina Ananiashvili was my third Raymonda. We first saw Ananiashvili in the 1980s, when the Bolshoi came to town with a slew of ballerinas. Ananiashvili was the youngest, and so leggy, linear, she was embraced as more western than the rest. In the last twenty years she's become an international star, guesting here and there, though recently she's settled in at ABT. Ananiashvili continues to wear her Bolshoi background lightly (she never had that eagle-has-landed Bolshoi swoop and drive), and this continues to be her charm. Now that she's older, there's a childlike, coloring-book quality to her dancing. All the steps are there, but mostly in outline, airily done, impulsive patches of color within. Ananiashvili can be quite brilliant—her allegro in *Raymonda* glittered—but she doesn't work deep in plié and it robs her of roundness, makes her seem a bit stick figure. Yet this too is part of her charm, that dash of naïveté, the way it simplifies, sweetens, her jet-set theatricality. When Ananiashvili dances with her longtime partner Julio Bocca they're like two old troupers taking their art, or the best that's left of it, to the provinces—except the province is New York City. And still they're irresistible. Is Ananiashvili a ballerina? Her fans, a formidable claque, would howl at the mere question. Certainly there's nothing exploratory about Ananiashvili's dancing, and it's not kinetically interesting, but the way she catches her own light—it's a late-day sun—and shines it into the audience, that too is power.

No one, however, had the resonance in *Raymonda* that came from a soloist only two years with ABT, Veronika Part. Trained at the Imperial School of the Mariinsky Theatre, Part was dancing ballerina roles with the Kirov by the late nineties. When the company brought its *Jewels* to the Met in 2002, she danced "Emeralds" as if born in its forest. Later that week, her Saturday matinee *Swan Lake* was epiphany: there were still depths in Odette. At that performance, the critic Don Daniels said New York hadn't seen such a *Swan Lake* since Makarova's. He was talking about something in Part's physical nature, her freedom within a phrase, a strength that allows her a further path. If a ballerina must show us something that we've never seen before—and I think she must—than Part is the most important ballerina dancing today. And she isn't even a principal.

Part never danced the lead in *Raymonda*, but stole the show as Henrietta, one of Raymonda's friends (the beautiful friend who may secretly dream of the convent). At ABT's opening night gala, an evening of razzle-dazzle, the *Raymonda* Act Two Pas de Sept took everyone by surprise, because of Part. She didn't seem to realize it was a gala. She was at a different party, the one for Raymonda. Her solo rolled out pianissimo, as when you sing softly outdoors and alone, allowing yourself a sudden syncopation, a flowering hold, a deeper low note (as in sinking to the floor) that returns you to a wider sky. Deeper, lower, lighter, higher, stronger, softer, stranger—Part's dynamic range is opulent, and her solo shivered with little graces, time-space undulations. The audience was silent, stunned, not the usual gala response where screams are the order of the evening, but the usual response to Part. She is commanding in every way.

Dance critics don't talk much about bodies anymore, or rather, female bodies. It seems to have been deemed politically incorrect, impolite, as if it's unfair to discuss something that can't be changed. But the body is where it all begins and Part's is one of the wonders of ballet today. Actually, I think she scares people. The beauty of her proportions aside (and feet bunheads dream on), Part does not conform to ballet's standard of sinewy thinness. She's 5 feet 8 inches, tall for a ballerina, and her figure has a nineteenth-century cadence, an hourglass allure. Her legs, long and straight as they are, boast grand-piano curves in the thigh and calf, not the cut muscles of a runner but planes rounded in rosewood. She has long arms set in wide shoulders, and this, coupled with her Russian training—that legendary calm at the clavicle, the Romanesque vaults in the port de bras—gives her enormous breadth and play above the bust, the reach of a huntress. She has a bosom, not big by civilian measure, but for ballet a downy décolletage—next to all those flat chests she's a little bit snowbound. And then the snow princess face: white white skin, black hair, a young Ava Gardner, a big white rose. She's completely voluptuous.

A little *too* voluptuous when she joined ABT in the fall of 2002. Part made her ABT debut at New York's City Center in the hallowed role of *Symphony in C*, second movement. The audience was packed with tout le monde, and the tone of the place was a mix of anticipation, admiration, and ill will (jealousies stir outside a company as well as within). Part had put on weight, and ABT did not have a partner to support her properly. Instead of borrowing a tall man from another company, and in a most unchivalrous manner, ABT threw her to the wolves with a reed of a cavalier. Part was heroic. No, she didn't have the freedom she needed in the middle register, but that lotus-blossom aplomb, the ivory-sceptor extension *en avant*, the pacific delicacy in the wrists and hands, the high horizon of the bust: one saw the endowments in relief, not the engine but the ice caps, and the vast poetic landscape spread before and beneath her.

By all accounts, hers included, it was a tough transition. All ballet companies are competitive, but where Kirov dancers have grown up together as family, coddled and coached the whole way, the ethic at ABT is sink or swim. Isolated by language, her outsider status, a spate of small injuries, her seriousness in rehearsal plus a tendency to tears, not to mention the usual resentments of rivals, Part was slow to climb, and ABT doled her out with an eyedropper. But artists draw strength from isolation, and Part's key solos were astonishments, Diaghilev's *étonnez-moi* meets Vreeland's "Give them what they never knew they wanted." Who'd have thought one could love the third shade in *La Bayadère*, the most tortured of three solo variations? Part took what usually looks like a dread physics test—all those delayed *développés* and dead stops in fifth—and made it seem a cat and mouse with moonbeams. Legato is her bowl of cream. And speaking of those leg extensions, correct, strong, long, they come up like a law of nature, almost animal, and stay like light. At intermission, a young dancer in the audience called Part's *développé* "3D," and she was right; it's not a step when Part does it, but a glory. Even in the heavily gowned, secondary role of *Romeo and Juliet's* Lady Capulet, Part found her way to a couplet. Opera glasses were trained on her hands, which had a Renaissance elegance, a painterly precision—pure theater. Part doesn't toss steps off, she takes the ballet in. As Queen of the Dryads in *Don Quixote*, in those swinging Italian fouettés, she seems to make an untouchable turret of that return perch in attitude, looking out the arched window, amber and amethyst, of her arm in high fifth.

"Veronika is never empty," said the great Kirov ballerina and now ABT coach, Irina Kolpakova, knocking a fist to her heart. "There is always more."

Finally, this spring at the Met, fit and slimmed in her fourth New York season with ABT, Part was moved into the spotlight. The ballet was *Mozartiana*, a company premiere for ABT, and the centerpiece of the company's Balanchine evening, an homage to the master in his centennial year. Choreographed in 1981, *Mozartiana* is Balanchine's last masterpiece, a ballet about reverence, dedication to an art one loves, and to the life-consuming requirements of such dedication—hence the four little girls, then the four big girls, then the ballerina. And yet audiences don't love this ballet. Perhaps the kaleidoscope Balanchine makes with the number four, symmetrically opening then closing space, is too mathematical a Mozart, too formal or distant a view. Perhaps the ballet-recital gradation—little, bigger, biggest—taps into a collective unconscious of childhood recitals long past and good riddance. Perhaps the ballet within the ballet—the superb pas de deux with its storm pitch of drama, its circling paths and tiny cliff—is too abstract. Or maybe it's the whisper of that black tulle veiled over white, the knowledge that no amount of love will hold us here, we must each leave in our time. Watching *Mozartiana*, it can feel as if Balanchine composed it not from the ground but from above, looking down on the stage. Suzanne Farrell, the woman on whom it was made, described the ballet with words from the Lord's Prayer: "on earth as it is in heaven."

Meanings knit up in *Mozartiana*. The bow/curtsy that ends every ballet class, an homage to the teacher and to the privilege of dancing ballet, is called révérence. It is but a deeper, more elaborate version of the bow that lives in the baroque (when ballet was born), a point made in *Mozartiana*'s third movement, the Menuet. Balanchine connects class to classicism, and like leaves or fruit falling drops that bow lightly, poignantly, all through the ballet. It's a little Mozartian world, chilly then sunny then trembling, built on the emotions of women and the inspiration of the one woman, the ballerina (and in his feeling for women, Mozart was right up there with Balanchine). The Gigue, always cast with a boyish virtuoso (in black satin knickers—the trouser role!), could be *Figaro*'s Cherubino singing of love's conundrums. And after all, the music itself is a révérence: Tchaikovsky orchestrated these Mozart melodies out of love for the great Amadeus.

Mozartiana is about endings and beginnings. Notice the steps. Skips, hops, jetés—schoolyard steps, tossed like seeds. And look at the way Balanchine gives first-year ballet steps to the ballerina, but sostenuto, almost deconstructing them, the way one must in the beginning to learn them. Those arabesque-passé-passés in the opening Preghiera (Prayer), like steps on stilts; the slow-motion *chaînés* in the ballerina's solos; the *échappés* done with a scissory half turn—these simple steps scaled greatly contain wisdom, a floating valediction, like late Matisse cutouts. The ballet *is* something to be scaled, and so the prayer at the beginning, the ballerina posed in a garden of little girls, is the invocation before the ascension. This ballerina must be big.

Maria Calegari, the former NYCB dancer and a rococo flame in the role herself, staged *Mozartiana* for ABT and chose three women for the lead: Ashley Tuttle, Nina Ananiashvili, and Veronika Part. Tuttle was miscast, too small literally and figuratively. Ananiashvili brought her usual charms to the role, and there were those who liked her *Mozartiana* best, no doubt because it was closer, superficially, to Farrell's. There are physical similarities between the two, for instance, the long legs with widening thighs. Also, both came to the role older, their plié shallower and so their dancing cooler, though Farrell, because of her spontaneity, was always dewy. Ananiashvili is not spontaneous. There were dead spots in her performance, seconds in which she had to wait to begin because she'd finished too soon, on the beat but off the wit. Farrell made even her flubs look witty.

Obviously, Farrell's performance of *Mozartiana* is the point of comparison. It was constructed to her strengths—that flying crane scale; her mysterious stamina; her playing with the music, teasing it with a head toss. When the ballet premiered Farrell was thirty-six, a dancer approaching the end of her career, just as Balanchine was nearing the end of his life (he died two years later). It was a time when Farrell's life-long extravagances—her almost religious commitment to dance, her whirlwind abandon—were less acts than inflections: two hip replacements were soon in her future. Balanchine gave Farrell sacred weight in the Preghiera with a series of reverential *temps liés* (a sliding through space in demi-plié, here with the hands pressed in prayer). The rest of the role, however, has a skimming brilliance, the hover and flash of a dragonfly. Balanchine had already acknowledged the physical change in Farrell. In 1980, for the muse figure she danced in *Robert*

Schumann's *"Davidsbündlertänze,"* he'd fashioned a solo of similar hovers and darts. And even as early as the celestial *Chaconne*, in 1976, the Farrell part is principally about pointe, heights, shooting-star extensions, all rays and flares, with plié receding, and the ache of adagio, its heavier cantilena line, virtually gone from her realm. So a leggy, skimming style warms the hearts of fans who want late-Farrell roles performed by late-Farrell types, which is to say with quixotic late-Farrell alignments (or is it limitations?). It's the treasured memory as judgmental ghost light.

I haven't seen every lead in *Mozartiana* since 1981, but I've seen many, and I've never seen one like Part's, which was monumental. She did it her way from the start, bringing that dynamic amplitude and lyric hearing to Balanchine's tricky simplicities. And Part's cameo glow—she's bonbon beautiful in her black satin bodice—it's crucial to a role in which She is Everything. In the Preghiera, Part was something of the captive princess grieving amid her court of little girls, and something of Mozart's Countess Almaviva, pouring her soul into "Porgi, amor," heartbroken, but why?

"I feel there's some secret in this ballet," Part told *Time Out* magazine in the week before her debut. "I haven't found the answer yet." Chinese proverb: "A bird does not sing because it has an answer. It sings because it has a song."

After the Preghiera the ballerina is offstage during the Gigue and Menuet. She returns for the Thème et Variations, a long back and forth between the ballerina and her cavalier, a dialogue that ends in an unusual pas de deux, flirtatious play that peaks heatedly, a bit Titania and Oberon, a touch of *Chaconne*, then ends on a thin ledge of repose, an aerie not quite of this world. It was in Part's solos that we began to see phenomenon unfettered, a complete integration of power and delicacy. Part dances in 360 degrees and you see it clearly in *Mozartiana*, where so many steps are cut from their moorings. So much dancing today looks *en face* even when it's not, as if framed for a flat screen. This is because dancers are concentrating on what happens to the front of the stage and ahead of their bodies; you'd never know there are eight fixed points on the stage, three of them to the rear. Part dances with her shoulders, bust, back, head, and hands, as well as legs and feet. She'll wing a *renversé* blindly behind and her whole being follows. She's not afraid of where her momentums will take her, those moment-to-moment displacements, and some of them are outrageous. A lunge into *relevé en arabesque* is a skydive from Heaven into a cloud of white tulle—white space she nests in. The moment is frightening in its force and in the pressure it puts on those long sapling feet that are sometimes soft, but it also feels pulled from her like poetry. Part brings her own gravity onstage.

And her own rules. It would be easy for Part to settle on portrait prettiness. And yet this dancer whose muscles seem fed by some luminous inner spring, and who needs that spring to support her breadth and length in body and limb, is willing to give us physical peril, plunges into risk, just as Farrell did. Some have called Part slow. Well, she's slow like a big cat with a terrific pounce. If anything, the word is *sloe*, the dark plum of the blackthorn—dancing that is rounded and full. Where Farrell's *Mozartiana* was a strand of sparkling recoveries, Part's is more maiden and minotaur, beauties sloe-ly unspooled. And if Farrell seemed to be lifting away from earth as if to follow Balanchine, Part is still reading this world, her body one with its curves and contours, still hearing its sad chthonic rumbles. It's that "more" Kolpakova spoke of. When Balanchine makes an existential game of *chaîné* turns on a diagonal, throwing a passé onto each pointe and slowing them down until they're a turning tightrope walk, Part plays another game. She doesn't wind down to a gawky ticktock like everyone else does (even Farrell), she creates a sensation: How slow can this go and not fall and still flow? I'll never forget those *chaînés*, like mist on still water.

We live in a time when strength has come to mean a buttoned-up performance, clean as a gymnastics routine, cool "doing" ever more two-dimensional, presentational, airtight. This is what people respond to in the dancing of Svetlana Zakharova, Sylvie Guillem: a whiplike dominatrix control that pushes you back in your seat in submission. But when you over-control you lose what is unknown, magical. Part is bucking every trend in ballet. She uses her strength to touch the precarious, to go where others can't or won't. And she shows us everything, making herself vulnerable (and pulling us forward for more). On a smaller scale, so does Roberta Marquez, a

South American who danced two *La Bayadère*s with ABT and proved, lest we forget, that a balance can be a living, breathing thing. The mysteries of ballet are bound up in its volumes, and artistry in its listening physical harmonics. Part began *Mozartiana* ravishing and ended a little ravished, because she was never not dancing. What more is there?

Swan Lake, of course. Part was awarded one performance, partnered by the young comer Marcelo Gomes, big-limbed, dark, and perfect for her. It was the most awaited casting of the season, and quite a different *Swan Lake* from the one Part danced with the Kirov in 2002. That was a performance of undertows, Part a recessive Odette, the momentums of the role caught in her breast and back, those elemental legs pulling away. In her ABT *Swan Lake*, Part revealed the heart that's been in lamb's wool these last two years. Here was an emotional Odette, passionately pitched, her narrative flights clear and momentous, and the delicacies, those trilling *entrechat-passés en arrière*, for instance, like water singing. When Odette first allows herself to lean back upon Siegfried's chest, Part's surrender is impetuous, tendriled, something between rest and wrest. You never forget she's trapped in feathers, in Von Rothbart's spell. And when Odette approaches Siegfried with a full circling swoop of the arms that pulls her up to pointe, Part powers a whoosh so huge we see the danger of her love—she actually startled Gomes, overwhelmed him. The supernatural size of her, it is the conjuring of the spell blowing through her, white rush and strange heart—Wingwraith. This is imagination, wild and precise, rehearsed and released, big, bigger, biggest. This is Veronika Part, making bliss of the art once again.

October 2004

Index

A

Acocella, Joan, 122
Acosta, Carlos, 109
Adams, John, 22
Afterimages, 3
Afternoon of a Faun (Robbins), 62
Ailey, Alvin, 3
L'Allegro, Il Penseroso ed il Moderato, 123–125, 127
Alton, Robert, 137
American Ballet Theatre (ABT), 15, 17–18, 22, 27, 31, 59–60, 73, 78–84, 86, 95, 109, 112, 116–117, 125–126, 132, 141–148, 150, 153
Americans We, 20
Ananiashvili, Nina, 145–146, 150
Anastasia, 38
Anderson, Leroy, 125
Angels in America, 10
Ansanelli, Alexandra, 139
Apollo, 14, 16, 18, 20, 99
Apollon Musagète (Stravinsky), 131
Appalachian Spring, 41–42, 46

L'Après-midi d'un Faune, (Mallarmé), 54, 100: Nijinsky, 91, 100
Arabesque, 91–92
Armitage, Karole, 21–25
Ashley, Merrill, 16
Ashton, Frederick, 3, 11–12, 17, 32–40, 74, 94, 126
Asnes, Andrew, 90
Astaire, Fred, 94, 102, 130
Asylmuratova, Altynai, 76, 105
Austen, Jane, 38–39
Avedon, Richard, 26
Ayupova, Zhanna, 105, 110

B

Bach, J. S., 62–63, 70, 93, 98, 128
Badchonim, 15
Bakst, Léon, 71
Balanchine, George, 3–4, 13–15, 18–19, 23, 25, 32–35, 38–40, 47–58, 60, 62, 65, 68–69, 71, 76–79, 82, 84–85, 89, 94, 96–101, 103–105, 107–108,

Index

110–113, 116, 120–122, 124, 126, 130–131, 133, 135, 138, 142, 144, 148–152
Ballet Review, 47, 72, 76, 85, 114, 123
Ballets Russes, 92, 104
Barak, Melissa, 95–96
Barraud, Henri, 55
Bartók, Béla, 55
Baryshnikov, Mikhail, 15, 18–19, 22, 26–31, 78–80, 103, 116, 124, 143
Bates, Ronald, 48
Bausch, Pina, 22
La Bayadère, 3, 78, 82–83, 107–110, 148, 153
Beach Birds, 97–98
Begichev and Geltser, 64
Bender, Gretchen, 10
Behemoth, 121
Berlin, Irving, 137
Bernstein, Leonard, 5, 60, 62–63
Besterman, Doug, 137
Billy the Kid, 78, 80
Bishton, Jamie, 29
Black Mountain College, 41
Bluebeard's Castle, 55
Bocca, Julio, 17, 82, 116, 146
Bolshoi Ballet, 38, 83, 145
Born to Be Wild: The Leading Men of American Ballet Theatre, 126
Bourne, Matthew, 67–69, 83, 115
Bowman, Benjamin G., 117
Brandenburg, 63
Brianza, Carlotta, 76
Brigadoon, 131

Britten, Benjamin, 38
Brooklyn Academy of Music (BAM), 7–9, 21–23, 25, 28, 42–43, 123, 126–127
BAMevent, 45
Brown, Tricia, 28
Brown, Zack, 144
Bruhn, Erik, 26
Buckle, Richard, 53
Bussell, Darcey, 32, 38
Byrne, David, 117

C

Caballé, Montserrat, 14
The Cage, 62
Cage, John, 41, 45
Calegari, Maria, 14, 150
Camelot, 144
Caplan, Elliot, 43
Cargo X, 43
Carnival of the Animals, 101
Carousel, 21, 131
Cascade, 88
The Catherine Wheel, 117
Cavanaugh, Michael, 117
Cecchetti, Enrico, 38
Chaconne, 151
Chausson, Ernest, 85
Chen See, Richard, 92
Chybowski, Michael, 126
Cinderella, 13, 15
Cinderella (Ashton), 34–37, 40
Clarke, Martha, 22
Cloven Kingdom, 88
Company B, 10, 89–90, 118
The Concert, 62

Index

Concerto Barocco, 98
Contact, 134–135, 138
Copeland, Roger, 42
Copland, Aaron, 80, 130
Coppélia, 71, 133
Corbin, Patrick, 90, 92, 128
Cordell, Fanchon, 142
Corella, Angel, 17, 20, 78–83, 109, 116
Le Corsaire, 79, 80, 82–83
Counterswarm, 122
Croce, Arlene, 3–4, 8, 33, 52, 120
Cunningham, Merce, 3, 28, 30, 41–46, 90, 97, 122

D

Dances at a Gathering, 62
Dance to the Piper, 130
Dandelion Wine, 89
Daniel, David, 95, 141
Daniels, Don, 114, 146
Danilova, Alexandra, 56
Davydov, Yury Lvovich, 65
The Death of Klinghoffer, 22
Debussy, Claude, 52–54, 91–92, 100
Delerue, Georges, 24
de Keersmaeker, Anna Teresa, 22, 30
De Luz, Joaquin, 132
de Mille, Agnes, 3, 42, 118, 130–132, 135–136, 139
Denby, Edwin, 2, 36, 59, 61, 81
Deuce Coupe, 116–117
de Valois, Ninette, 33

Diaghilev, Serge, 92, 104, 106, 148
Diamond Project, 39
"Diamonds," 47–49, 52, 54, 56–58, 98, 111–112
Dido and Aeneas, 124
Le Dieu Bleu, 92
Don Quixote, 16, 110, 133, 148
Donaldson, Walter, 138
Double Feature, 133–134, 136
Doubrovska, Felia, 104
Dream Girls, 128
Dudinskaya, Natalia, 14
Dunn, Douglas, 42–43
Dybbuk, 62–63

E

Egtvedt, Kristi, 92
Einstein on the Beach, 21–23
The Elements, 15, 20
The Elizabethan Phrasing of Albert Ayler, 22
"Emeralds," 48–50, 52–55, 57, 146
Endangered Species, 21
Esplanade, 87
Eugene Onegin, 66
Everlast, 117

F

Facade: An Entertainment with Poems by Edith Sitwell, 126
Fadeyev, Andrian, 109
Falconer, Ian, 100–101
Fancy Free, 59–61

Index

Farrell, Suzanne, 14, 22–23, 52, 54, 56–58, 113, 149–152
Fauré, Gabriel, 49, 53–54, 111
Fiddler on the Roof, 59
Fiends Angelical, 89
The Figure in the Carpet, 13–14
La Fille mal gardée, 38
Finley, Karen, 9
Fonteyn, Margot, 14, 36–37, 71, 75, 80, 82
Forsythe, William, 24, 38
Foursome, 123, 127
The Four Temperaments, 35, 51, 98, 124, 133
Franck, César, 12
Frederick Ashton and His Ballets, 37
Funny Papers, 90

G

Gantz, Jeffrey, 3
Gates, Jr., Henry Louis, 8
Gergiev, Valery, 106
Gilman, Howard, 28
Giselle, 27, 76, 82, 107, 109, 138, 143
Glass, Philip, 22
Glazunov, Alexander, 144
Gloria, 121, 127
Gold, Tom, 139
Goldberg Variations, 62
Golub, Irina, 110
Gomes, Marcelo, 109, 153
Gong, 125
Graham, Martha, 3, 6, 41–43, 46, 87–88, 92, 130–131, 139
The Great Russian Dancers, 26

Greenberg, Neil, 11
Greer, Fergus, 28
Greskovic, Robert, 57
Guillem, Sylvie, 111, 152
Gumerova, Sofia, 110–111

H

Hammerstein, Oscar, 131
The Hard Nut, 67
Harvard Theatre Collection, 72
Hawkins, Erick, 29, 31, 41
Hayden, Melissa, 85–86
Helpmann, Robert, 36
Herrera, Paloma, 15–17, 83, 109, 141
Holding On to the Air, 52
Holmes, Anna-Marie, 144
Houston Ballet, 15, 109
Huot, Jesse, 117
Hynninen, Airi, 85

I

If You Couldn't See Me, 28
Les Illuminations, 38
Imperial School of the Mariinsky Theatre, 143, 146
Installations, 43, 45
Interplay, 61, 63
Ivanov, Lev, 68–69, 98
Ivesiana, 101
Ives, Songs, 62

Index

J

Jaffe, Susan, 17
Jardin aux Lilas, 82–85, 94
Jerome Robbins' Broadway, 60
Jewels, 47–50, 52–58, 107,
　110–111, 113, 133, 146
Joel, Billy, 115, 117
The Joffrey Ballet, 33, 116
Joffrey, Robert, 3
Jones, Bill T., 4, 7–10, 23
Journey of a Poet, 29

K

Kael, Pauline, 4, 61
Karinska, Barbara, 48, 50, 54
Karsavina, Tamara, 103
Kavanagh, Julie, 32
Kawakubo, Rei, 44
Kay, Hershy, 137
Kaye, Danny, 137
Kaye, Nora, 132
Kelly, Glen, 137
Kent, Allegra, 101
Kent, Julie, 17–18, 82, 132
Kimball, Roger, 5
The King and I, 59–60
Kirkeby, Per, 69
Kirkland, Gelsey, 14, 142–143
Kirov Ballet, 72, 103, 105
Kisselgoff, Anna, 75
Kirstein, Lincoln, 3, 13–14, 33
Kistler, Darci, 57–58
The Kitchen, 11
Koleda Folk Ensemble, 122
Kolpakova, Irina, 14, 75, 148, 152

Korsuntsev, Danila, 110
Kowroski, Maria, 15–16
Kramer, Hilton, 5
Kushner, Tony, 10
Kylian, Jiri, 15

L

Last Look, 127
*Last Supper at Uncle Tom's Cabin/
　The Promised Land*, 9
Laurents, Arthur, 5
La Valse (Ashton), 33, 35
La Valse (Balanchine), 35
The Leaves Are Fading, 18
Le Clercq, Tanaquil, 56
Lerner and Loewe, 144
Letter to the World, 41
Liebeslieder Walzer, 120–121
Lifar, Serge, 20
Lifeforms, 45, 97
Ligeti, Gyorgy, 100
Lincoln Center Festival, 36
Lincoln Center Library, 142
Lobenthal, Joel, 90, 142
Lohengrin, 64
Lopatkina, Uliana, 76, 106–107
Loring, Eugene, 80, 130
Ludlow, Conrad, 47

M

MacMillan, Kenneth, 33, 36, 38
Maeterlinck, Maurice, 49, 52–55
Makarova, Natalia, 68, 103,
　142–143, 146
Makhalina, Yulia, 105–106

Malakhov, Vladimir, 17–19, 79, 81
Mallarmé, Stéphane, 54, 91, 100
Manon, 38, 82
Marquez, Roberta, 152
Martins, Peter, 15, 18, 24, 69, 95, 100, 111, 120, 133–134, 138
Mason, Francis, 47
Mayerling, 38
McBride, Patricia, 51, 58
McKenzie, Kevin, 83, 144
McKerrow, Amanda, 17, 132
Mejia, Paul, 56
Men's Piece, 116
Merce Cunningham: The Modernizing of Modern Dance, 42
Metamorphosis, 29
Meunier, Monique, 69
Mezentseva, Galina, 105
Miami City Ballet, 58
A Midsummer Night's Dream, (Mendelssohn), 71: Balanchine, 18, 49, 99, 133
A Midsummer Night's Dream, (Shakespeare), 49, 124
The Mollino Room, 22
Monumentum Pro Gesualdo, 96
Monumentum/Movements, 96
Morris, Mark, 8–9, 15, 27, 67, 120–129
Movements for Piano and Orchestra, 96
Movin' Out, 115, 117–119
Mozart, Amadeus, 71, 149, 151
Mozartiana, 113, 148–153
Murphy, Gillian, 132, 145
Musical Offering, 92
The Music Man, 134, 138

N

Neary, Patricia, 51
Nelson, Gene, 135–136
New Love Song Waltzes, 120
New York City Ballet (NYCB), 15–16, 32–33, 38–39, 47–48, 60, 62, 69, 78–79, 95, 99, 103, 120, 132, 142
Next Wave Festival, 21, 28, 42
Nichols, Kyra, 15, 57–58
Nijinsky, Vaslav, 26, 62, 91–93, 103
Nixon in China, 22
Noseda, Gianandrea, 72
Not-About-AIDS-Dance, 11
The Nutcracker, 67, 108, 133
Nureyev, Rudolf, 18–19, 26, 36, 46, 80, 103

O

O'Day, Kevin, 15, 116
The Office, 122
Oh, You Kid!, 90
Oklahoma!, 21, 131, 134–135, 138
On the Town, 59–60
On Your Toes, 133
O Rangasayee, 121
Orpheus, 3
Osmolkina, Ekaterina, 114

P

Parkinson, Elizabeth, 117
Part, Veronika, 107, 110–111, 146–148, 150–153

Index

Pavane pour une infante défunte, 39–40
Pavlenko, Daria, 107, 110–112
Pavlova, Anna, 71, 103
Pelléas et Mélisande, 49, 52–53, 55
El Penitente, 41
Perl, Jed, 23
Perrault, Charles, 55, 70
Peter Pan, 59
Petipa, Marius, 33, 49, 70–76, 80, 98–99, 107–108, 143
Piazzola Caldera, 89
Pillar of Fire, 131–132
Polyphonia, 100–102
Ponomarev, Vladimir, 108
Porter, Michael, 123
Poznansky, Alexander, 66
The Predators' Ball: Hucksters of the Soul, 21–25
The Prince of the Pagodas, 36, 38
Private Domain, 91
The Prodigal Son, 16, 98, 104
Proia, Alexandre, 141
Promethean Fire, 128
Purcell, Henry, 124
Push Comes to Shove, 78, 80, 116

R

Rachlis, Kit, 3
Ravel, Maurice, 35–36, 39, 133
Raymonda, 143–146
The Red Shoes, 1, 14
Reitz, Dana, 30
Remote, 29
Resurrection, 126
Reyes, Xiomara, 145

Robbins, Jerome, 3–5, 18, 59–63, 100, 118, 130, 133, 139, 142
Robert Schumann's "Davidsbündlertänze," 40
Roberts, Keith, 117
Rodeo, 132
Rodgers, Richard, 126, 131
Romeo and Juliet, 17, 19, 38, 62
Rondo, 45
The Royal Ballet, 36
Royal Ballet School, 39
Royal Danish Ballet, 69
"Rubies," 48–51, 54, 56–57, 111
Russian Imperial Ballet, 33
Ruzimatov, Farukh, 106
Ryan, Thomas Jay, 23

S

Le Sacre du Printemps, 91
Le Sacre du Printemps (The Rehearsal), 91
Sadler's Wells Ballet, 33
Saint-Saëns, Camille, 101
Salle, David, 22–23
Samodurov, Viacheslav, 109
San Francisco Ballet, 125
Sandpaper Ballet, 125
Scenario, 43–45
Scènes de Ballet, 100
Schéhérazade, 92
Scherbakov, Vasili, 109, 114
Schiller, Johann, 39
Schoenberg, Arnold, 57, 132
Scholl, Tim, 72–73
School of American Ballet (SAB), 15, 63, 79, 95, 100, 104, 142

Index

Schorer, Suki, 47, 55, 104
Schumann, Robert, 40, 126–127, 151
Scotch Symphony, 105
Secret Muses: The Life of Frederick Ashton, 32–33
Secret Pastures, 7
Selya, John, 116–117
Septet, 28, 30–31
Serenade, 15, 34
Sergeyev, Nikolai, 72
Shearer, Moira, 14, 37
Shylock, 49
Sibley, Antoinette, 37
Sizova, Alla, 75
Slavonic Dances, 39–40
Slaughter on Tenth Avenue, 126, 133
The Sleeping Beauty, (Tchaikovsky), 70–71: Ashton, 35, 71; Martins, 133; Petipa, 17, 33, 36–38, 49, 60, 70–76, 98, 106–108, 124, 144; Sergeyev, 72, 76, 105
Smakov, Gennady, 26
The Snow Maiden, 65
Sologub, Natalia, 110, 114
Something Lies Beyond the Scene, 126
Sondheim, Stephen, 5
Stars and Stripes, 133
St. Denis, Ruth, 30
Stepping Stones, 15
Stiefel, Ethan, 17–19, 78–83
Still/Here, 4, 8–10, 12, 23
The Stories of the Great Ballets, 1
Stravinsky, Igor, 49–50, 62, 91, 96, 111, 131, 133

Stroman, Susan, 132–139
Strukov, Vadim, 114
Stuart, Meg, 29–30
Swan Lake, (Tchaikovsky), 56, 64–66, 68, 70–71: Balanchine, 68–69; Baryshnikov, 27; Bourne, 67–69, 83, 115; Martins, 69, 133; McKenzie, 83, 153; Petipa-Ivanov, 17, 38, 49, 51–52, 54, 56, 68; Sergeyev, 113–114, 146
La Sylphide, 83
Les Sylphides, 1
Sylvia, 1, 71
Symphonic Variations, 11–12, 17, 35–36, 38
Symphony in C, 16, 57, 76, 107, 147

T

Taming of the Shrew, 78
Taper, Bernard, 34, 99
Taylor, Paul, 3, 10–11, 41, 87–93, 97, 118, 122, 127–128, 137
Tchaikovsky, Pyotr Ilyich, 17, 49, 52, 54, 58, 64–66, 68–72, 74, 76–77, 82, 103, 108, 111, 133, 149
Telemann Overture Suite in E Minor, 95
Terekhova, Tatiana, 105
Tharp, Twyla, 15, 20, 27, 30, 80, 115–119, 123
Theme and Variations, 79, 82, 105, 143
Three Epitaphs, 88
Torke, Michael, 69

161

Index

Tracey, Margaret, 16, 57
Trilling, Lionel, 39
Trusnovec, Michael, 92, 127
Tudor, Antony, 3, 84–86, 94, 130–132
Tuttle, Ashley, 82, 117–118, 150
2 & 3 Part Inventions, 63

U

Undine, 53–54, 65, 70
Union Jack, 133
Unspoken Territory, 30

V

V, 127–128
Vaganova Academy, 143
Vaganova, Agrippina, 103, 107
Valse Fantaisie, 18
Variations Serieuses, 102
Vasiev, Makhar, 72, 106
Vaughan, David, 36–37
Vera-Ellen, 137
Verdy, Violette, 49–50, 53–55, 57–58
Vienna Waltzes, 112
Vikharev, Sergei, 76
Villella, Edward, 47–48, 51, 56, 58, 62
Vinogradov, Oleg, 105–106
Viola, Lisa, 90, 92, 128
Vishneva, Diana, 76, 107, 110–111
Vivaldi, Antonio, 121
Volkov, Solomon, 69, 103
Vsevolozhsky, Ivan, 70, 72–74

W

Wagner, Richard, 64–65, 71, 124
Wagner, Robin, 137
Walton, William, 126
Webern, Anton, 93
Weese, Miranda, 57
Western Symphony, 133
West Side Story, 4, 59–62, 124
Wheeldon, Christopher, 36, 39–40, 99–102
Whelan, Wendy, 57, 101
White, Diana, 16
White Oak Dance Project, 27–28, 31, 124
Wise, Robert, 4
Who Cares?, 16, 133, 137
Wiley, Roland John, 64–65, 71, 75
Wilson, Robert, 22, 25, 62
Windows, 45
Woetzel, Damian, 138
The Word, 122
Wuorinen, Charles, 69

Z

Zakharova, Svetlana, 76, 111, 152
Zane, Arnie, 7, 9
Zelensky, Igor, 17, 20